T0229299

INTERVENTIONAL CARDIOLOGY CLINICS

www.interventional.theclinics.com

Editor-in-Chief

MATTHEW J. PRICE

Transradial Angiography and Intervention

January 2020 • Volume 9 • Number 1

ELSEVIER

1600 John F. Kennedy Boulevard • Suite 1800 • Philadelphia, Pennsylvania, 19103-2899

http://www.theclinics.com

INTERVENTIONAL CARDIOLOGY CLINICS Volume 9, Number 1
January 2020 ISSN 2211-7458, ISBN-13: 978-0-323-73311-3

Editor: Stacy Eastman
Developmental Editor: Donald Mumford

Interventional Cardiology Clinics (ISSN 2211-7458) is published quarterly by Elsevier Inc., 360 Park Avenue South, New York, NY 10010-1710. Months of issue are January, April, July, and October. Subscription prices are USD 209 per year for US individuals, USD 495 for US institutions, USD 100 per year for US students, USD 209 per year for Canadian individuals, USD 590 for Canadian institutions, USD 100 per year for Canadian students, USD 296 per year for international individuals, USD 590 for international institutions, and USD 150 per year for international students. To receive student/resident rate, orders must be accompanied by name of affiliated institution, date of term, and the *signature* of program/residency coordinator on institution letterhead. Orders will be billed at individual rate until proof of status is received. Foreign air speed delivery is included in all *Clinics* subscription prices. All prices are subject to change without notice. **POSTMASTER:** Send address changes to *Interventional Cardiology Clinics*, Elsevier Health Sciences Division, Subscription Customer Service, 3251 Riverport Lane, Maryland Heights, MO 63043. **Customer Service: Telephone: 1-800-654-2452** (U.S. and Canada); **1-314-447-8871** (outside U.S. and Canada). **Fax: 1-314-447-8029. E-mail: journalscustomerservice-usa@elsevier.com (for print support); journalsonlinesupport-usa@elsevier.com (for online support).**

Reprints. For copies of 100 or more of articles in this publication, please contact the Commercial Reprints Department, Elsevier Inc., 360 Park Avenue South, New York, NY 10010-1710. Tel.: 212-633-3874; Fax: 212-633-3820; E-mail: reprints@elsevier.com.

CONTRIBUTORS

EDITOR-IN-CHIEF

MATTHEW J. PRICE, MD
Director, Cardiac Catheterization Laboratory,
Division of Cardiovascular Diseases, Scripps
Clinic, La Jolla, California, USA

EDITOR

BINITA SHAH, MD, MS
Assistant Professor of Medicine, Associate
Director of Research, Cardiac Catheterization
Laboratory, Division of Cardiology
(Interventional Cardiology), Department of
Medicine, New York University School of
Medicine and the New York VA Harbor
Healthcare System, New York, New York, USA

AUTHORS

ELIE AKL, MD
Department of Medicine, Division of
Cardiology, McMaster University, Hamilton,
Ontario, Canada

AHMAD ALSHATTI, MD
Department of Medicine, Division of
Cardiology, McMaster University, Hamilton,
Ontario, Canada

AMIT P. AMIN, MD, MSc
Cardiovascular Division, Barnes-Jewish
Hospital, Center for Value and Innovation,
Washington University School of Medicine, St
Louis, Missouri, USA

MAURICIO G. COHEN, MD, FACC, FSCAI
Professor of Medicine, Cardiovascular
Division, Department of Medicine, University
of Miami Miller School of Medicine, Miami,
Florida, USA

RHIAN E. DAVIES, DO, MS
Division of Cardiology, University of
Washington, Seattle, Washington,
USA

MARVIN ENG, MD
Center for Structural Heart Disease, Henry
Ford Hospital, Detroit, Michigan, USA

ALEXANDER C. FANAROFF, MD, MHS
Assistant Professor of Medicine, Division of
Cardiology, University of Pennsylvania,
Philadelphia, Pennsylvania, USA

TIBERIO FRISOLI, MD
Center for Structural Heart Disease, Henry
Ford Hospital, Detroit, Michigan, USA

DIOGO C. HAUSSEN, MD
Assistant Professor, Departments of
Neurology, Neurosurgery, and Radiology,
Emory University School of Medicine, Grady
Memorial Hospital, Marcus Stroke and
Neuroscience Center, Atlanta, Georgia, USA

SANJIT S. JOLLY, MD, MSc
Department of Medicine, Division of
Cardiology, McMaster University, Population
Health Research Institute, Hamilton, Ontario,
Canada

KATHLEEN E. KEARNEY, MD
Division of Cardiology, University of
Washington, Seattle, Washington, USA

PRIYANK KHANDELWAL, MD
Assistant Professor, Department of
Neurosurgery and Neurology, Rutgers
University, Newark, New Jersey, USA

SAMUEL M. LINDNER, MD
Cardiovascular Division, Washington
University School of Medicine, Barnes-Jewish
Hospital, St Louis, Missouri, USA

JAMES M. McCABE, MD
Division of Cardiology, University of
Washington, Seattle, Washington, USA

CHRISTIAN A. McNEELY, MD
Cardiovascular Division, Washington
University School of Medicine, Barnes-Jewish
Hospital, St Louis, Missouri, USA

BRETT M. MILFORD, DO
Interventional Cardiology Fellow,
Cardiovascular Division, Department of
Medicine, University of Miami Miller School of
Medicine, Miami, Florida, USA

RAUL G. NOGUEIRA, MD
Professor, Departments of Neurology,
Neurosurgery, and Radiology, Emory
University School of Medicine, Grady
Memorial Hospital, Marcus Stroke and
Neuroscience Center, Atlanta, Georgia, USA

WILLIAM O'NEILL, MD
Center for Structural Heart Disease, Henry
Ford Hospital, Detroit, Michigan, USA

SAMIR B. PANCHOLY, MD
Division of Cardiology, The Wright Center for
Graduate Medical Education, Scranton,
Pennsylvania, USA

GAURAV A. PATEL, MD
Division of Cardiology, The Wright Center for
Graduate Medical Education, Scranton,
Pennsylvania, USA

PRATIT PATEL, MD
Fellow, Department of Neurosurgery, Rutgers
University, Newark, New Jersey, USA

TEJAS M. PATEL, MD
Division of Cardiology, Apex Heart Institute,
G-K Mondeal Business Park, Ahmedabad,
Gujarat, India

SRIDEVI R. PITTA, MD, MBA
Cox Health System, Interventional
Cardiologist, Associate Professor of Clinical
Medicine, University of Missouri School of
Medicine, Springfield, Missouri, USA

ABHIRAM PRASAD, MD
Professor of Medicine, Department of
Cardiovascular Medicine, Mayo Clinic,
Rochester, Minnesota, USA

SUNIL V. RAO, MD
Professor of Medicine, Division of Cardiology,
Duke Clinical Research Institute, Duke
University, Durham, North Carolina, USA

MOHAMMED K. RASHID, MD
Department of Medicine, Division of
Cardiology, McMaster University, Hamilton,
Ontario, Canada

JORDAN G. SAFIRSTEIN, MD
Director, Department of Cardiology,
Transradial Intervention, Morristown Medical
Center, Morristown, New Jersey, USA

SANJAY C. SHAH, MD
Division of Cardiology, Apex Heart Institute,
Ahmedabad, Gujarat, India

RAJESH V. SWAMINATHAN, MD
Associate Professor of Medicine, Division of
Cardiology, Duke Clinical Research Institute,
Duke University, Durham, North Carolina,
USA

PEDRO A. VILLABLANCA, MD, MSc
Center for Structural Heart Disease, Henry
Ford Hospital, Detroit, Michigan, USA

CONTENTS

 Video content accompanies this article at http://www.interventional.theclinics.com.

> Over the past 2 decades, radial artery access has increasingly become the standard approach for coronary angiography and intervention. Compared with femoral arteries, transradial access is associated with better hemostasis. Transradial access has increased patient preference, facilitates early ambulation, and is cost-effective. An important limitation of transradial access is access site failure, and it carries a crossover rate of 3% to 7% in randomized prospective trials comparing radial with femoral artery access among experienced operators. Crossover rates for failed primary radial artery access can be reduced with ultrasonography guidance and increased familiarity with alternative access sites in the wrist.

> Transradial artery access (TRA) is associated with reduced bleeding risk, length of stay, costs, and increased patient satisfaction. Approximately one-third of TRA failures are due to lack of guiding catheter support. Catheter selection and engagement technique are crucial for obtaining good-quality angiograms and successfully completing percutaneous coronary intervention. The maneuvers required for catheter manipulation and coronary engagement differ between TRA and transfemoral arterial access. One of the advantages of TRA is the ability to use a universal catheter, saving time, radiation, and contrast. This review discusses practical learning points to improve operator understanding of catheter selection and coronary engagement technique.

> Considerable evidence supports transradial angiography and intervention in patients with acute coronary syndrome, with an emphasis on decreasing major bleeding and access site vascular complications. Patients undergoing invasive treatment are at greatest risk of bleeding and have the most to gain. The radial advantage has consistently been shown to translate into reduced mortality in pooled data analyses. The benefits of transradial access have been demonstrated across the acute coronary syndrome spectrum and in both sexes. A radial-first strategy should be the default approach and continuous efforts should be made to increase operator expertise of transradial access in these patients.

This article highlights the advantages and disadvantages of transradial arterial (TRA) access for a variety of presentations including acute coronary syndromes; cardiogenic shock; unprotected left main, heavily calcified coronaries; bifurcations; and chronic total occlusions. It includes techniques for overcoming challenges of using TRA access, including spasm and the need for larger bore guides. In addition, the authors review the use of ultrasound for access, percutaneous hemodynamic support via axillary approach, and tips and tricks to performing right heart catheterizations from the antecubital vein.

Peripheral vascular intervention (PVI) improves quality of life and reduces major adverse limb events in patients with peripheral arterial disease. PVI is commonly performed via the femoral artery, and the most common adverse periprocedural event is a vascular access complication. Transradial access for PVI has the potential to reduce vascular access complications and improve patient outcomes. Further study is needed to elucidate the risks of stroke, acute kidney injury, and radiation exposure in the setting of transradial PVI. As transradial access for PVI progresses, it will be important to build the evidence base along with procedural experience.

The transradial approach has emerged as the preferred alternative to the traditional transfemoral approach owing to the increased evidence of its safety and efficacy. The field of structural heart disease is rapidly evolving; however, periprocedural complications related to access site remain a major determinant of morbidity and mortality. The transradial approach as primary or secondary access site in structural heart interventions like transcatheter aortic valve replacement, balloon aortic valvuloplasty, alternative access, alcohol septal ablations, paravalvular leak, valve snaring, coronary protection, and ventricular septal defect is feasible, safe, with lower vascular complications and high procedural success.

 Video content accompanies this article at http://www.interventional.theclinics.com.

Trans-radial approach (TRA) has been used in cardiac and peripheral interventional radiology practices for decades, because of safety and patient comfort. There is interest in TRA in the cerebrovascular field, with potential to replicate benefits over trans-femoral approach. TRA is technically more challenging and has a learning curve, which hinders its use as the first-line approach; however, as more neuro-interventionalists embrace TRA, techniques are being optimized simultaneously for supra-aortic vessel catheterization. This article describes advantages, patient selection, conventional and distal radial access, and detailed techniques of trans-radial catheterization for diagnostic angiography, as well as cerebrovascular interventions and its current limitations.

Transradial access has increased in utilization and has been shown to be superior compared with transfemoral access. Although infrequent, several transradial access site-related complications occur. By understanding potential mechanisms related to these complications, several prevention and treatment strategies can be implemented to mitigate adverse outcomes.

This article summarizes the data comparing radiation exposure and contrast use between transradial and transfemoral cardiac catheterizations. It also reviews the important features that may predict access site failure and crossover. In addition, it reviews the concept of ergonomics in the catheterization laboratory and how clinicians can improve the transradial approach.

This review summarizes the impact of transradial access for cardiac catheterization and percutaneous coronary intervention related to patient satisfaction, patient safety, and health care costs. In studies comparing transradial versus transfemoral approach, transradial access causes less bleeding and less vascular access site complications and provides a mortality benefit in patients with acute coronary syndromes. Transradial access improves patient satisfaction related to site tolerability by reducing pain and discomfort, and facilitating early ambulation with reduced length of stay. Taken in total, the existing randomized and observational data strongly support radial access for improved safety, patient satisfaction, and significant cost savings.

TRANSRADIAL ANGIOGRAPHY AND INTERVENTION

FORTHCOMING ISSUES

April 2020
Updates in Peripheral Vascular Intervention
Herbert D. Aronow, *Editor*

July 2020
Renal Disease and Coronary, Peripheral and Structural Interventions
Hitinder Gurm, *Editor*

RECENT ISSUES

October 2019
Hot Topics in Interventional Cardiology
Matthew J. Price, *Editor*

July 2019
Transcatheter Mitral Valve Repair and Replacement
Matthew J. Price, *Editor*

April 2019
Updates in Percutaneous Coronary Intervention
Matthew J. Price, *Editor*

RELATED SERIES

Cardiology Clinics
Cardiac Electrophysiology Clinics
Heart Failure Clinics

THE CLINICS ARE NOW AVAILABLE ONLINE!

Access your subscription at:
www.theclinics.com

PREFACE

Radial Access and Beyond: The Future of Cardiovascular Interventions May Run Through the Arm

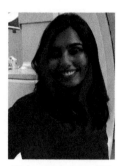

Binita Shah, MD, MS
Editor

This is an exciting time in the radial world. While we spent the last decade or so determining the benefits of and optimizing radial artery access in coronary angiography and percutaneous coronary intervention, the future pushes access in the arm to the realms of mechanical hemodynamic support devices, peripheral interventions, structural interventions, and neurointerventions. In this issue, our experts take the reader through the tips and tricks to radial, ulnar, and distal radial access and coronary cannulation, followed by the contemporary role of radial artery access in acute coronary syndromes and then detail the technical aspects of accessing the arm for both support devices and noncoronary interventions. The issue rounds out with a discussion on how to manage complications that may arise from accessing the arm through to optimization of radial access in terms of patient satisfaction, health care economics, and ergonomic tips for operator success. We hope our readers will gain not just information on additional tips and tricks that may help their everyday but also a vision for what can be done to potentially improve outcomes beyond just coronary interventions.

Binita Shah, MD, MS
Division of Cardiology
(Interventional Cardiology)
Department of Medicine
New York University
School of Medicine
New York VA Harbor
Healthcare System
423 East 23rd Street
Room 12023-W
New York, NY 10010, USA

E-mail address:
binita.shah@nyumc.org

Intervent Cardiol Clin 9 (2020) ix
https://doi.org/10.1016/j.iccl.2019.10.001
2211-7458/20/© 2019 Published by Elsevier Inc.

Accessing the Wrist
From Data to Tips and Tricks

Sridevi R. Pitta, MD, MBA[a,*], Abhiram Prasad, MD[b]

KEYWORDS

- Transradial access • Transulnar access • Transfemoral access • Left radial artery access
- Distal radial artery access • Ultrasound guided access • Coronary artery disease
- Percutaneous coronary intervention

KEY POINTS

- Over the past 2 decades, radial artery access has increasingly become the standard approach for coronary angiography and intervention.
- Compared with femoral arteries, transradial access is associated with better hemostasis because of its easy compressibility with reduced vascular complications.
- Transradial access has increased patient preference, facilitates early ambulation, and is cost-effective.
- An important limitation of transradial access is access site failure, and it carries a crossover rate of 3% to 7% in randomized prospective trials comparing radial with femoral artery access among experienced operators.
- Crossover rates for failed primary radial artery access can be reduced with ultrasonography guidance and increased familiarity with alternative access sites in the wrist.

 Video content accompanies this article at http://www.interventional.theclinics.com.

INTRODUCTION

Since the introduction of transradial artery access (TRA) by Campeau 3 decades ago, there has been a paradigm shift with an increased uptake of TRA for cardiovascular angiography and interventions worldwide.[1–5] However, TRA has several limitations because of the small caliber of the artery, which may limit device selection; high frequency of spasm; presence of radial artery anomalies; and postprocedural occlusion, which may preclude future usage of same artery.[6–9] Even with improved devices and techniques, access site crossover remains a concern and occurs in up to 7% of patients.[10,11] Appreciating different alternative approaches to TRA, including distal radial artery access (DRA) and transulnar artery access (TUA), increases

options for both operators and patients. This article reviews the technical aspects of TRA and the evidence regarding feasibility and safety of alternative wrist access sites.

TRANSRADIAL ACCESS

TRA has increasingly become a standard approach for cardiovascular angiography and intervention (class I recent European guidelines) and is overwhelmingly used worldwide. In patients with acute coronary syndrome, TRA reduces net adverse clinical events through reduction in major bleeding and all-cause mortality.[1,12,13] TRA also leads to improved quality-of-life measures, is strongly preferred by patients, and is associated with reduced hospital costs compared with transfemoral artery access (TFA) for coronary

Disclosure: The authors have no conflicts of interest.
[a] Cox Health System, University of Missouri School of Medicine, 3800 S National Avenue, Suite # 700, Springfield, MO 65807, USA; [b] Department of Cardiovascular Medicine, Mayo Clinic, 200 First Street, Rochester, MN 55905, USA
* Corresponding author.
E-mail address: pittas@health.missouri.edu

angiography and percutaneous coronary intervention (PCI).[14] A radial-first approach is strongly recommended with a graduated level of center and operator experience. Choice of right radial access (RRA) or left radial access (LRA) is per operator preference.

TECHNIQUE FOR TRANSRADIAL ARTERY ACCESS

Patient Selection

Although a radial-first approach should be encouraged for all comers depending on operator and center experience, TRA should be the preferred approach and is beneficial in patients with therapeutic anticoagulation, thrombocytopenia, morbid obesity, multiple comorbidities, heart failure symptoms, orthopedic injuries, and cognitive impairment.[12,15] Relative contraindications to TRA include patients needing radial artery for bypass conduit, dialysis fistula, vaso-occlusive disease (eg, Raynaud, Takayasu, thromboangiitis obliterans), and complex subclavian and brachial anatomy. RRA and LRA approaches for angiography have similar feasibility.[16] RRA is preferred because of operator comfort, whereas LRA offers advantages for patients with grafts, short stature, elderly (aged >75 years), and those with less subclavian tortuosity. LRA is also favored by operators early in the transition from TFA to TRA because of familiarity with catheter cannulation of the coronary arteries. Common reasons for crossover from RRA to LRA or TFA include small-caliber artery or radial artery occlusion (RAO), tortuosity, calcification, or spasm.[17,18] Disadvantages of LRA include application in patients with a large abdominal circumference, patient orthopedic conditions that may make supination for an unknown duration of the procedure difficult, and operator discomfort associated with flexion of the back.

Preprocedural Assessment

An Allen test or Barbeau test is performed to confirm dual arterial circulation to the hand and intact palmar arch system. However, patients undergoing TRA with normal versus abnormal preprocedural Allen test showed no difference in grip strength, thumb capillary, or incidence of hand ischemia. Noninvasive testing does not predict adverse outcomes and should not be used for access site triage (ie, abnormal Allen or Barbeau should not preclude TRA). Reverse Allen or Barbeau helps to identify an occluded radial artery filling with retrograde collaterals.[19,20] Good practice includes assessment of radial artery patency before discharge and at the first postprocedural visit (**Figs. 1** and **2**).

Patient Setup

Safe and successful TRA requires appropriate setup. For RRA, a platform that provides support for the access site, wires, and catheters is preferable (**Fig. 3**). Several arm boards available on the market allow external rotation of the arm and support wrist flexion. To minimize radiation exposure, radial operators should position the accessed arm close to the patient's torso. LRA requires the left elbow to be supported by pillows or newer support devices while the arm is brought over to the patient's right side so that it is closer to the right femoral region (**Fig. 4**).[21–25]

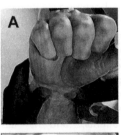
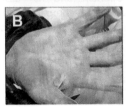
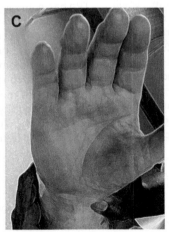
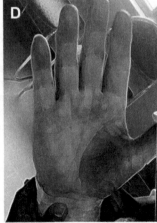

Fig. 1. Modified Allen test. (*A, B*) Palpate radial and ulnar arteries and obliterate both with the thumbs and fingers of both hands, followed by clenching the fist repeatedly until palm blanches white. (*C*) Then open the palm and release the ulnar pulse. Time to reappearance of palm color is 7 seconds (normal Allen) and abnormal if takes longer for return of palm color or no return (see Fig. 1). (*D*) Inverse allen test to assess patency of radial artery and performed similar to modified allens test except for release of radial artery.

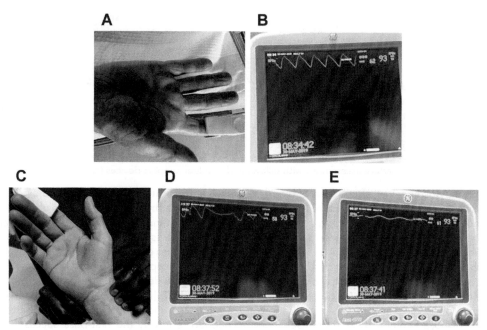

Fig. 2. Alternative Allen test (Barbeau test) includes modified Allen test and finger plethysmography. (*A, B*) Sensor to the thumb confirming normal tracing of pulse oximeter. (*C, D*) Releasing the ulnar artery and immediate return of tracing pulse oximeter confirms presence of collaterals. (*E*) Abnormal tracing suggests poor collaterals.

Access Technique

The ideal site for radial artery puncture is 2 cm to 3 cm proximal to the flexor crease of the wrist. Single-wall puncture or double-wall puncture is operator dependent. Modified Seldinger technique involves puncture of the anterior wall of the radial artery, followed by flow of arterial blood from the needle hub with introduction of the guidewire and sheath into the radial artery. Accessing more proximally is not recommended because the radial artery may be difficult to palpate beneath the forearm muscles and postprocedure hemostasis can be difficult, with a resultant increased risk of developing a hematoma. Accessing more distally (closer to the wrist joint) can result in perforation of the reticular ligament of the joint, and minor movements of the wrist can change the compression pressure. Seldinger technique involves entering the anterior wall of the radial artery followed by advancement of the Angiocath further

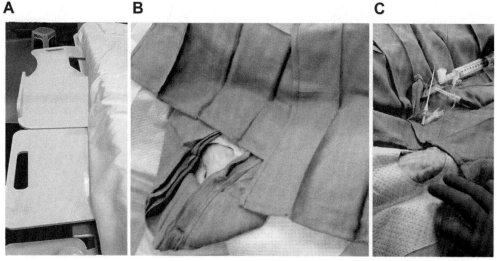

Fig. 3. Right radial artery access prep and setup. (*A*) Right radial setup using arm board. (*B*) Forearm supinated and wrist hyperextended at the site of puncture. (*C*) Arm positioned parallel to the table.

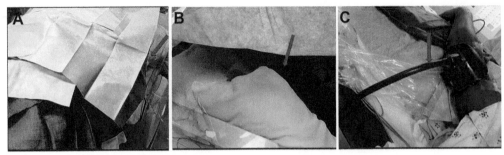

Fig. 4. (A–C) Left radial artery access prep with pillows and shoulder support devices (arrows).

through the posterior wall after a flash of blood is first visible at the hub of the Angiocath. The needle is removed and the Angiocath is then gradually withdrawn until pulsatile flow is seen at the hub. The Seldinger technique for TRA is associated with shorter time to gaining access and higher success rates on first attempt compared with the modified Seldinger technique (Figs. 5 and 6). The incidence of access site bleeding complications, as well as RAO, are comparable between Seldinger and modified Seldinger techniques. Palpation-guided TRA is associated with a crossover rate to femoral artery access on up to 7.6% with experienced operators. Ultrasonography guidance, particularly in patients with shock, weak pulse, or hypotension, improves arterial access success.[10,11,26–28]

Ultrasonography Guidance

Ultrasonography guidance facilitates precise cannulation of vessels regardless of anatomic variation, which can increase procedural success. In the United States, 48.8% of operators never use ultrasonography and only 4.4% use ultrasonography in more than 50% of cases.[1] Ultrasonography-guided TRA is associated with short learning curve and uses equipment that is readily available in most hospitals. Comparative studies of palpation-guided and ultrasonography-guided TRA (RAUST [Radial artery access with Ultrasound] trial) shows that the number of attempts needed is lower, the first-pass success rate is higher, and the time to access is shorter with ultrasonography guidance.[26] Point-of-care ultrasonography is affordable and easy to use in assisting in accurate vascular access (Fig. 7, Video 1). If ultrasonography-guided TRA is obtained, a 0.36-mm (0.014-inch) wire may be used if resistance is encountered.[29,30]

Sheath

Use the lowest profile of sheath to minimize trauma and spasm. Radial sheaths with tapered edge and hydrophilic coating allow smooth

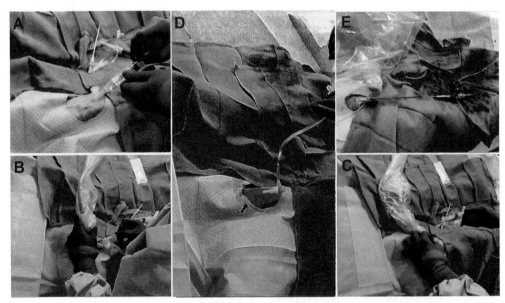

Fig. 5. (A–E) Right radial artery access. (A) Small amount of local anesthesia. (B) Ultrasound guided radial artery access. (C, D) Successful sheath insertion. (E) Followed by successful advancement of cornary catheters.

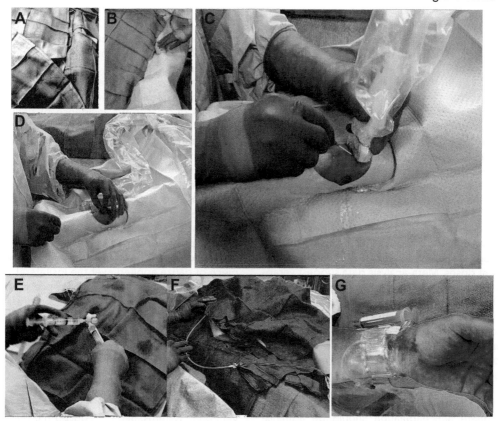

Fig. 6. Left radial artery access and hemostasis. (*A–D*) Accessing the left radial artery using ultrasound guidance. (*E, F*) Left arm propped with support and brought to the right side. (*G*) Hemostasis using TR band and Hemostatic patch.

insertion of the sheath and reduce the incidence of radial artery spasm. There is no impact of sheath length on incidence of RAO or spasm.[31,32]

Pharmacology

Pharmacologic agents for consideration include analgesics, antispasmolytics, and anticoagulants. Pain management during TRA is important

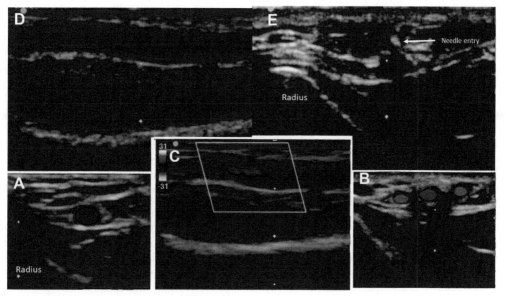

Fig. 7. (*A–E*) Ultrasonography-guided access.

because it reduces anxiety, discomfort, and associated vasoconstriction.[33,34]

Antispasmolytics

Radial artery spasm can be minimized with use of vasodilators. Data support the use of pretreatment with sublingual nitroglycerin 1 to 5 minutes before access. Spasmolytic agents can be also used intraprocedurally after sheath insertion, with each catheter exchange, and before sheath removal. Most operators use calcium channel blockers and/or nitroglycerin.[35–37] Verapamil is the most widely used calcium channel blocker; other dihydropyridine agents have reportedly been used and there is little evidence to suggest interclass difference with similarly potent doses. Meta-analysis data suggest verapamil 5 mg with or without nitroglycerin (200–400 μg) is the most effective spasmolytic agent.[38] In patients with hypotension, inferior myocardial infarction with right ventricle involvement, extremely low ejection fraction, or severe aortic stenosis, vasodilators should be used with caution.

Anticoagulation

Adequate anticoagulation should be administered in patients undergoing TRA procedures. Recommended regimens include intra-arterial or intravenous 50 units/kg or 5000 units in patients without contraindications to heparin. Patients with heparin-induced thrombocytopenia may receive bivalirudin 0.75 mg/kg bolus for diagnostics and bolus followed by infusion at 1.75 mg/kg/h for PCI.[39–41] Alternative anticoagulants, such as bivalirudin or enoxaparin, with comparative doses have been shown to have similar efficacy to unfractionated heparin in the prevention of RAO. In patients with therapeutic oral anticoagulant levels, use of additional adjunctive heparin is still needed to prevent RAO.[42]

Hemostasis

Achieving hemostasis after TRA may be less difficult compared with TFA. The radial artery is a much smaller artery than the femoral artery and, because of its superficial location, it is easier to apply direct pressure to the access site to achieve hemostasis. Although applying direct pressure is easier with the radial artery, occlusion of the radial artery is an important concern with TRA. The operator applying the hemostasis band should not apply flow-limiting compression, but should maintain patent hemostasis. Absence of radial artery flow during compression represents a strong predictor of RAO. Typically, the radial band can be loosened 30 minutes after diagnostic procedures and 90 to 120 minutes after interventional procedures. Preservation of antegrade arterial flow while maintaining hemostasis decreases the incidence of early occlusion (12% compressive vs 5% patent; $P<.05$) and late occlusion (7% compressive vs 1.8% patent; $P<.05$) and, as such, is superior to traditional compression of the radial artery. Consider the use of prophylactic ipsilateral ulnar artery compression to reduce RAO rates, compared with standard patent hemostasis (0.9% vs 3%; $P = .0001$). A radial hemostatic band is positioned over the radial sheath entry site. Next, a compression band is placed over a piece of gauze applied over the ipsilateral ulnar artery in the Guyon canal, and, once plethysmography confirms ulnar artery compression, the radial sheath is removed and the TR Band is inflated using the patent hemostasis protocol.[8,43,44]

Using strategies to shorten the duration of radial artery compression with the use of a topical hemostatic pad in conjunction with a radial band such as the TR Band (Terumo Interventional Systems, Japan) reduced the duration of radial artery compression in a nonrandomized case series.[45,46] A StatSeal disc (StatSeal Advanced, BioLife, Sarasota, FL), comprising a topical hydrophilic polymer and potassium ferrate compound, forms an occlusive seal on contact with even a small amount of blood. The StatSeal protocol includes a compression device and the StatSeal Advanced disc in place. Air from the balloon is removed to decrease the volume to 5 cm³ within 20 minutes for diagnostic procedures and 60 to 90 minutes for PCI procedures. After an additional minimum 20 minutes, the hemostasis balloon is slowly deflated in a stepwise manner until fully deflated. If hematoma or bleeding develops at any time during the protocol, the balloon should be reinflated to the prior volume, left in place for at least 20 minutes, and then the deflation protocol resumed (**Fig. 8**) (Video 2).

DISTAL RADIAL ARTERY ACCESS

A novel technique using the DRA for access via the anatomic snuffbox was first described by Kiemeneij[47] in 2017 in a series of 62 patients. Since then, the experience with the technique has been described by a few other operators. DRA is now more inclusive and describes puncture of the radial artery, not just at the anatomic snuffbox above the scaphoid but anywhere

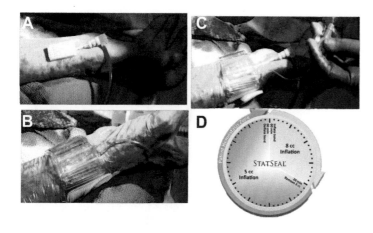

Fig. 8. (*A–C*) Transradial hemostasis using TR Band and hemostatic patch. (*D*) Hemostatic patch protocol (StatSeal disc, StatSeal Advanced, BioLife). (*Courtesy of Biolife, Sarasota FL.*)

along the distal radial artery trajectory across the carpal bones. Advantages of DRA include increased patient comfort with dorsal positioning of the hand, operator ergonomics when used for left-sided access, and absence of venous compression by the compression device, which has the potential for causing venous stasis in the hand and fingers. Additional potential advantages compared with conventional TRA include preservation of antegrade flow, minimization of hand ischemia because access is obtained distal to the superficial palmar arch, and faster hemostasis because of the smaller caliber of vessels beyond the bifurcation. For patients in professions dependent on right hand dexterity (eg, mechanics, musicians), left DRA can be advantageous.[48–50]

Feasibility

A retrospective review of 408 patients showed that successful access was obtained in 99.5% of the DRA cases and in 99% among TRA conventional cases. However, the access site crossover rate in the DRA group was ultimately 2%. Mean access time was 7.3 minutes longer with DRA than conventional TRA (7.3 minutes vs 5.2 minutes), but hemostasis was obtained faster with DRA compared with conventional TRA (104.6 ± 40.6 minutes vs 178.6 ± 68.1 minutes; $P<.001$).[51,52]

Safety

Another single-center review of 200 consecutive patients undergoing left DRA reported postprocedure puncture site complications among 15 patients (7.9%), which included minor hematomas 14 (7.4%) and arterial dissection 1 (0.5%). There was no occurrence of DRA occlusion, perforation, pseudoaneurysm, or arteriovenous fistula.[52,53]

Anatomy

The anatomic snuffbox is a small triangular space along the dorsal radial aspect of the wrist, made evident when the thumb is extended. The margins include the tendons of the abductor pollicis longus and the extensor pollicis brevis muscles laterally, medially by the tendon of the extensor pollicis longus muscle, the base is formed by the distal margin of the retinaculum of extensor muscles, and the vertex is formed by the attachment of the tendons of extensor pollicis longus and extensor pollicis brevis muscles, respectively. The distal radius, scaphoid, trapezium, and the base of the first metacarpal bone form the foundation of this triangular area. The roof is formed by the skin and superficial fascia, which contain the cephalic vein and superficial branch of the radial nerve. The DRA passes deeper through the anatomic snuffbox (lateral aspect of the dorsum of the wrist). Distally, the radial artery continues as the deep palmar branch and joins the distal part of the ulnar artery, forming the deep palmar arch of the hand. The artery in the anatomic snuffbox is distal to the superficial palmar branch of the radial artery, which joins the superficial palmar arch. Multiple collateral vessels communicate between the superficial and deep palmar arches. Hence occlusion of the DRA in the anatomic snuffbox causes less ischemia because antegrade flow is maintained through the superficial palmar arch and the communicating collaterals (**Fig. 9**).[51]

TECHNIQUE FOR DISTAL RADIAL ARTERY
Prep

The right hand is pronated to a comfortable position with the anatomic snuffbox facing upward. The patient is positioned with the arm in a neutral position and a small towel to hold for

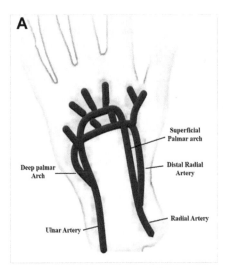
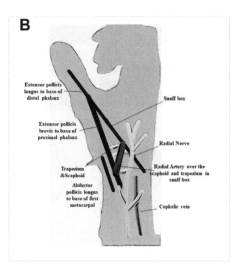

Fig. 9. (A) Blood vasculature of the hand. (B) Anatomy; relationship of distal radial artery to the surrounding tendons and vessels in the snuffbox. (Adapted from [A] Aoi S, Htun WW, Freeo S, et al. Distal transradial artery access in the anatomical snuffbox for coronary angiography as an alternative access site for faster hemostasis. Catheter Cardiovasc Interv. 2019; with permission; and [B] Vilela FD, Boechat e Salles JA, Cortes LA, et al. Distal transradial access in the anatomical snuffbox for coronary angiography and aortography. J Anat Physiol Stud 2017;1(1):1–3; with permission.)

comfort and also to open the dorsal area separating the thumb and the first finger (Fig. 10, Video 3). The left hand is positioned at the left groin with support underneath the left elbow and the arm gently flexed at the shoulder with homemade support methods (pillows and blankets) to adduct the instrumented arm or with dedicated DRA support devices such as the Cobra Board device (TZ Medical), which prevents arm drift during left radial artery procedures (see Figs. 4C and 14A).[48]

Access

The DRA is palpable between the bony prominence of the thumb and first finger. Arterial puncture may be performed using palpation or ultrasonography guidance. In the original series by Kiemeneij,[47] despite the superficial position over the bony prominence, the distal radial was found to be too weak to attempt puncture in approximately one-quarter of cases, which is more frequent than with conventional TRA. DRA vessel diameter in the anatomic snuffbox was

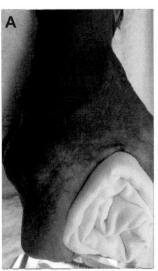
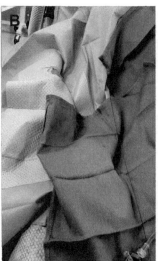
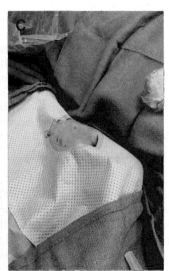

Fig. 10. (A) Right arm with small towel to hold separating the thumb and the first finger. (B, C) Right hand dorsal side facing up in a comfortable position.

significantly smaller (2.6 ± 0.5 mm) than that of the proximal radial artery (PRA) at the conventional puncture site (3.1 ± 0.4 mm). The difference in vessel diameter between the DRA and PRA was 0.5 ± 0.4 mm.[54] The smaller mean distal radial lumen diameter in women compared with men (2.1 vs 2.4 mm respectively; $P<.01$) makes access slightly more challenging in women.[54,55]

Palpation

Access is obtained at the site of the strongest pulse, and access may be obtained at the dorsum of the hand rather than the anatomic snuffbox because it is superficial and easily compressed between first and second metacarpal bones. Some operators prefer bare needles because of concerns of through-and-through puncture at the snuffbox touching the periosteum of bones, which can be painful. The needle should be angled at 30° to 45° from lateral to medial. The needle should be directed at the strongest pulse and can access the dorsum of the hand, distal to the tendon of extensor pollicis longus muscle where it is more superficial than the snuffbox and easily compressed against the metacarpal bones.

Ultrasonography Guidance

Ultrasonography aids in assessing the size and location of the artery, which, in turn, increases success rates and minimizes vasospasm related to multiple punctures. Ultrasonography aids in selecting appropriate sheath size and excluding

cases in which the artery is too small. In addition, venous access can be obtained at the same time as arterial access. Using short-axis and long-axis views, along with color flow, can be helpful (Fig. 11, Video 4).[54,55]

After the access with either bare needle or standard double puncture using a 20-gauge needle, an appropriately sized sheath is introduced (4–6-Fr thin-walled sheath over a soft-tipped J-shaped 5.3-mm [0.21-inch] wire). The wire should not be forced because any resistance encountered could be caused by deflection into the side branch or dissection plane. Fluoroscopy should be used to determine the wire path and to navigate tortuosity and branches in case of resistance (Fig. 12). A small skin incision can be made to prevent kinking of the sheath at the insertion site, because the skin is thicker and harder than in the forearm. Most DRA failures were caused by inability to thread the guidewire after encountering resistance despite good backflow in the needle (Figs. 13 and 14). Vasodilators and anticoagulation should be administered, similar to conventional TRA. After access has been secured, the patient's arm can be moved to a comfortable position for both the patient and operator. The procedure can be completed using the standard diagnostic catheters and guides, similar to conventional TRA. Continuous photoplethysmography monitoring using the ipsilateral thumb or fingers should be performed throughout the procedure and after completion (Video 5).

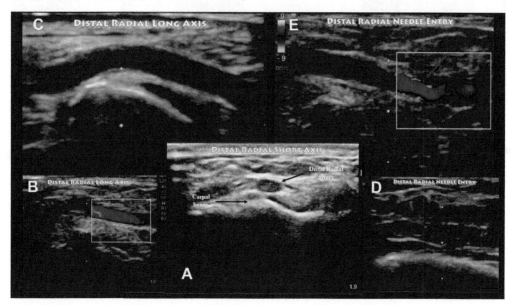

Fig. 11. Ultrasonography-guided access. (A–C) Short-axis view of the distal radial artery Superficial nature and long-axis views of the distal radial artery with and without color above the carpal bones (*arrows*). (D, E) Short-axis and long-axis views showing needle entry of the artery, seen as echogenic structure (*arrow*).

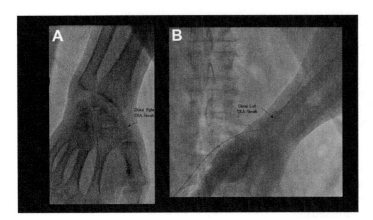

Fig. 12. (*A*, *B*) Radiograph showing access point at the wrist joint with wire navigation under fluoroscopy.

Hemostasis

After completion of the procedure, hemostasis is obtained using the TR Band (Terumo Medical, Japan). The TR Band is modified for DRA by removing the hard-plastic plate component to allow it to conform to the distal access puncture site (**Fig. 15**). Dedicated distal radial hemostatic devices (PreludeSYNC, Merit Medical) are also now available. The authors have adapted a modified StatSeal protocol (**Fig. 16**, Video 6).

Conclusions

DRA is feasible and safe for coronary angiography and interventions. It provides an alternative to conventional TRA with possible faster

hemostasis time and lower rate of artery occlusion and other complications. Because of its smaller caliber, DRA requires a steeper learning curve, and ultrasonography visualization is recommended. This new technique needs further exploration and larger randomized comparison studies to definitively show the potential advantages.

ULNAR ARTERY ACCESS

Arterial access from the wrist is most commonly obtained from the radial artery. Despite the advantages of TRA, limitations include crossover rate to the femoral approach in as many as

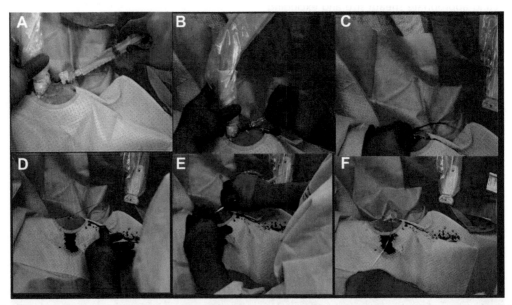

Fig. 13. Access of the right distal radial. (*A*) Liberal amount of lidocaine injected at the access site. (*B*) Ultrasonography-guided angled needle entry and Angiocath. (*C*) Slow withdrawal of the Angiocath for pulsatile flow. (*D–F*) Placement of wire and exchange for 6-Fr Terumo slender hydrophilic sheath. ([*D–F*] *Courtesy of* Terumo, Tokyo, Japan.)

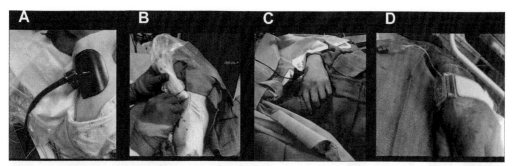

Fig. 14. Left radial access. (*A*) Left shoulder support device with palm over the left groin. (*B, C*) Ultrasonography-guided access of the left distal radius from the right side of the table. (*D*) Hemostasis with TR Band and StatSeal. ([*D*] Courtesy of Biolife, Sarasota FL.)

7.6% of cases using palpation guidance,[29,30] RAO in 3% to 6%, radial artery spasm around 10%, and high anatomic variants and loops in 5% of cases. Transulnar artery access (TUA) may be considered an alternative approach in cases with high probability of TRA failure or complications caused by small radial diameter, radial stenosis/calcification, tortuosity, and other anatomic issues.

Feasibility

A prospective, randomized, multicenter, parallel-group study involving 902 patients (the AURA of ARTEMIS study) showed higher crossover rates in the TUA group and remained inferior to TRA with a difference of 26.34% (95% confidence interval [CI], 11.96%–40.69%;

$P = .004$). Limitations of this study were that operators had adequate TRA experience but no specific training in TUA.[56] A nonrandomized observational report (AJULAR study) comparing 410 patients undergoing TUA versus TRA coronary procedures (performed by a single experienced operator who performs >150 TRA procedures per year and at least 50 TUA procedures) found no difference in procedure time, fluoroscopy times, and cannulation attempts. However, these parameters were higher with TUA versus TRA in other reports that included inexperienced operators.[57,58] A systematic review and meta-analysis of 6 randomized controlled trials showed no difference in the incidence of major adverse cardiovascular events (MACE), arterial access time, fluoroscopy time,

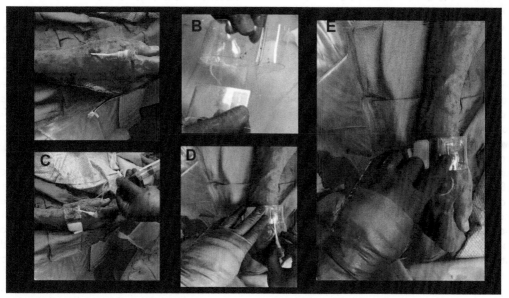

Fig. 15. (*A*) Sheath in the distal radius. (*B*) Plastic sheet removal from the TR Band. (*C*) Application of the TR Band with 8 to 10 mL of air balloon inflation. (*D, E*) Removal of the sheath and confirming hemostasis. (*Courtesy of* Biolife, Sarasota FL.)

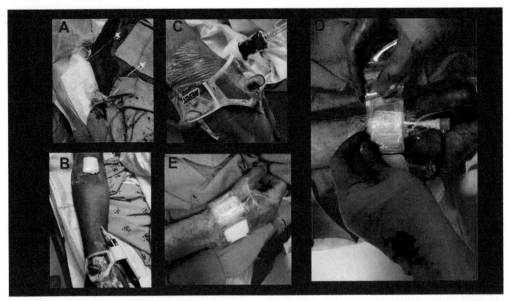

Fig. 16. (A) Using hemostatic patch with TR Band and dedicated devices (Prelude). (A–C) A 6-Fr sheath in the cephalic vein for right heart catheterization and 6-Fr sheath in the right distal radius, followed by manual pressure to remove the venous sheath in the cephalic vein and dedicated device for DRA. (D, E) StatSeal with TR Band for DRA. (Courtesy of Biolife, Sarasota FL.)

and contrast load between patients undergoing TUA versus TRA.[59] TUA requires specific skills to be learned even for experienced TRA operators.[60] Despite the available data and lower rate of anatomic variations, loops, tortuosity, and adrenergic receptor rates that result in spasm, adoption of TUA has been low, likely because of the deeper location of the ulnar artery compared with the radial artery, and its proximity to the ulnar nerve.

Safety

Complication rates are low and comparable between TUA and TRA when performed by experienced operators. In the intention-to-treat analysis the AURA of ARTEMIS study, the composite primary end point of access site crossover, MACE, and major vascular events of the arm at 60 days was significantly higher in the ulnar arm (42.2%) compared with the radial arm (18%); however, this was largely driven by higher crossover rate. Further meta-analysis of 6 trials showed no statistically significant difference in the incidence of MACE between patients who underwent TUA and TRA catheterization (odds ratio, 0.90; 95% CI, 0.65–1.25). Complications associated with access, including hematoma formation (n = 6 trials), pseudoaneurysm, and arteriovenous fistulae formation (n = 5 trials), were investigated in a total of 5276 patients, with no difference in these complications noted

between the two groups. There is evidence to support the safe use of the ulnar artery as an alternative to the radial artery for access for cardiac catheterization.[56,59,61]

Anatomic Aspects

The ulnar artery originates 5 to 7 cm distal to the elbow and is a major branch of the brachial artery. It runs along the medial portion of the forearm, adjacent to the ulnar nerve in the distal forearm. The artery courses medially to the pisiform bone, covered by various muscles and tendons in the forearm, dividing into 2 branches after crossing the transverse carpal ligament and pisiform bone. The 2 branches form the superficial palmar arch (40%–80% complete) fed by the superficial ulnar medially and superficial branch of radial laterally. The deep palmar arch is formed (99% complete) by the deep palmar branch of ulnar artery (medially) and radial artery (laterally) (Fig. 17A). The anterior interosseous artery arises proximally along the ulnar artery and is a predominant source of collaterals when there is an RAO. The ulnar artery is most superficial and best palpated proximal to the flexor skin crease at the wrist, but still deeper compared with the radial artery (Fig. 17B). The ulnar nerve runs medial and parallel to the ulnar artery in the distal forearm, and both are encased by the restrictive Guyton canal in the wrist. Hence arterial puncture should start on

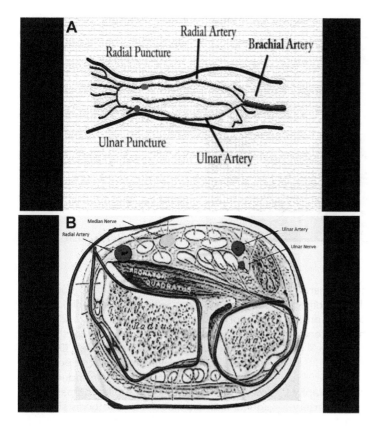

Fig. 17. (*A*) Forearm vascular structure and access site for ulnar artery. (*B*) Relationship of the ulnar artery to surrounding anatomic structures. ([A] *Adapted from* Khan S. Ulnar Access for Catheterization and Intervention: When and how radial operators should consider transulnar access as an alternative to transfemoral access. Cardiac Interventions Today. 2017.; with permission.)

the lateral side of the ulnar artery to minimize pain and spasm.[62]

TECHNIQUE TO ULNAR ARTERY ACCESS
Technical Aspects
Performing a routine Allen test been challenged by many operators for both TRA and TUA, because access is feasible and safe even in the presence of abnormal Allen/Barbeau test.[20] Modified Allen test is performed by occlusive pressures to the radial and ulnar arteries while the hand is elevated and closed tightly for about 30 seconds to obstruct the blood flow to the hand. While the hand is still elevated, it is opened, and release of ulnar pressure alone should restore color to the hand. A small prospective study of 131 patients by Vassilev and colleagues[63] suggested that a palpable ulnar artery and normal modified Allen test is associated with low access site complication rates. TUA technique is similar to TRA. Use the smallest-diameter sheath to minimize risk of arterial injury and patient discomfort, and conscious sedation to mitigate arterial spasm. The arm and forearm should be positioned comfortably in a supinated and hyperextended position to accentuate the site of maximal pulse prominence. Lower success rates are attributed to deeper location of the ulnar artery, proximity of the artery around or below the tendon of the muscle flexor carpi ulnaris, absence of good bone base as in the radial artery, and proximity to ulnar nerve potentially making puncture painful.[63]

Puncture Site
Similar to TRA, right ulnar artery is preferred to the left for operator convenience. The left ulnar artery may be preferred in patients with known prior coronary artery bypass surgery with a patent left internal mammary artery graft or potentially complex coronary intervention, based on TRA data.[60,64]

Palpation Guided
Arterial puncture should be from the lateral aspect of the ulnar artery to reduce the likelihood of pain caused by ulnar nerve injury, because the nerve lies medial to the ulnar artery. Cannulation needs to be close to the wrist skin crease because of the inability to compress the artery 5 cm or more proximal to the crease. After infiltration of local anesthesia approximately 1 cm proximal to the

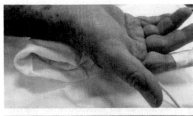
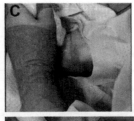
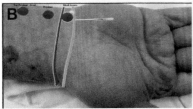
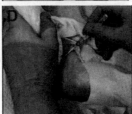

Fig. 18. (A) Hyperextension of the wrist for ulnar artery prominence and palpation. (B) Optimal location of ulnar artery access along the lateral side of the artery in the wrist fold. Proximal locations are not ideal and produce more complications. (C, D) Real-time ultrasonography-guided access.

flexor skin crease, the artery is punctured where it can be best palpated using the modified Seldinger technique. A higher puncture site proximal to the wrist is associated with hematomas (Fig. 18).

Ultrasonography Guidance

In a study of preprocedural ultrasonography among 2344 patients, the mean ulnar artery diameter was 1.8 mm in men and 1.6 mm in women. Arterial abnormalities were observed in 9.8%[65] (high bifurcations, loops, occlusions). Ultrasonography measurements show that the ulnar artery was larger than the radial artery in 6.5% of patients and of similar size in 58.5%. Real-time intraprocedural ultrasonography helps to understand anatomy and anomalies, which improves access site success[30] (Fig. 19, Video 7). Moreover ultrasonography guidance allows the selection of appropriate sheath size by measuring vessel diameter and hence reducing spasm and improving the overall success of arterial access from the wrist with reduced crossover rates to a secondary access site.[30] Puncturing can also be done with a bare needle, with an anterior puncture technique using a 21-gauge needle (cephalad angle 60°–70° to the wrist fold proximal to the pisiform bone). Once the needle enters the lumen, a soft-tipped 0.46-mm (0.018-inch) guidewire is introduced followed by the sheath with a dilator. Spasmolytic agents and anticoagulation protocols similar to TRA can be used. This step is followed by advancement of a 0.89-mm (0.035-inch) J wire or a 1.5-mm J-tip 0.89-mm hydrophilic wire (Fig. 20).

Hemostasis

Achieving appropriate hemostasis after TUA and preventing ischemic complications is very important. Graded compression with the minimal effective occlusive pressure using commercially available hemostasis devices used for TRA is recommended after ulnar sheath removal. The duration of compression should be the shortest time possible while allowing

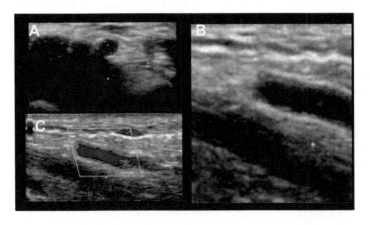

Fig. 19. (A) Real-time ultrasonography images showing the short-axis view of the ulnar artery surrounded by tendon and muscles, and with poor bony support. (B, C) Long-axis view of the ulnar artery and color imaging of the long axis.

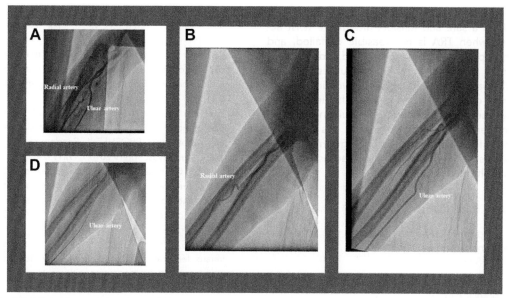

Fig. 20. (A) Angiogram showing radial artery spasm and ipsilateral ulnar artery being patent and followed by TUA. (B, C) Angiogram showing radial artery tortuosity and kinks and failed navigation. Ipsilateral ulnar artery is patent with minimal tortuosity. (D) Successful ulnar artery access followed by 0.89-mm (0.035″) wire for navigation of catheters.

ulnar distal flow to minimize the likelihood of arterial occlusion. The compression balloon is aligned with the ulnar artery, as for TRA. Simultaneous hemostasis of both the radial and ulnar arteries may be performed using 2 balloon compression devices in a failed TRA approach followed by a successful TUA approach (Fig. 21).[8] Ischemic injuries have been reported as uncommon in TUA. This finding could be attributed to the reported larger caliber of the ulnar artery and dual blood supply to the hand by the radial artery.[66,67]

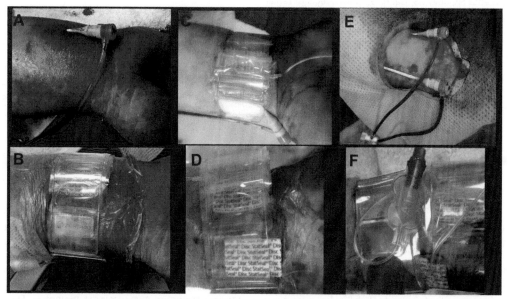

Fig. 21. (A, B) Ulnar artery access with 6-Fr slender sheath and hemostasis with hemostatic patch with TR Band. (C, D) Dual access for failed radial access with postprocedural hemostasis with 2 patches and single TR Band. (E, F) Radial access sheath proximally and ulnar access sheath closer to the wrist fold. Hemostasis with 2 patches and 2 TR Bands. (*Courtesy of* Biolife, Sarasota FL.)

Summary

TUA is a safe and feasible alternative wrist access, when TRA is not feasible or failed, and when performed by experienced radial operators.[68] To maintain a higher success rate of wrist-based interventions while avoiding the potential complications, operators should consider the use of ultrasonography guidance.[64] The long-term safety and efficacy of this approach needs further investigation in larger multicenter cohorts before it can be endorsed as the standard alternative to TRA.

SUPPLEMENTARY DATA

Supplementary data related to this article can be found online at https://doi.org/10.1016/j.iccl.2019.08.009.

REFERENCES

1. Shroff AR, Fernandez C, Vidovich MI, et al. Contemporary transradial access practices: results of the second international survey. Catheter Cardiovasc Interv 2019;93(7):1276–87.

2. Romagnoli E, Biondi-Zoccai G, Sciahbasi A, et al. Radial versus femoral randomized investigation in ST-segment elevation acute coronary syndrome: the RIFLE-STEACS (Radial Versus Femoral Randomized Investigation in ST-Elevation Acute Coronary Syndrome) study. J Am Coll Cardiol 2012;60(24):2481–9.

3. Mehta SR, Jolly SS, Cairns J, et al. Effects of radial versus femoral artery access in patients with acute coronary syndromes with or without ST-segment elevation. J Am Coll Cardiol 2012;60(24):2490–9.

4. Rao SV, Hess CN, Barham B, et al. A registry-based randomized trial comparing radial and femoral approaches in women undergoing percutaneous coronary intervention: the SAFE-PCI for Women (Study of Access Site for Enhancement of PCI for Women) trial. JACC Cardiovasc Interv 2014;7(8):857–67.

5. Goel PK, Menon A, Mullasari AS, et al. Transradial access for coronary diagnostic and interventional procedures: consensus statement and recommendations for India: advancing Complex CoronariES Sciences through TransRADIAL intervention in India - ACCESS RADIAL: clinical consensus recommendations in collaboration with Cardiological Society of India (CSI). Indian Heart J 2018;70(6):922–33.

6. Pitta SR, Sharma R. Radial artery occlusion after transradial cardiac catheterization: tips on prevention and management. 2018. Available at: http://www.scai.org/press/detail.aspx?cid=87d2ca49-a67f-406f-bf88-6de659dea01a#.XRM3a3dFyUk.

7. Pitta SR, Sharma R. 2017. Available at: http://www.scai.org/QITTip/entrapped-radial-sheath-stepwise-algorithm-to-untr.

8. Pancholy SB, Karuparthi PR, Gulati R. A novel non-pharmacologic technique to remove entrapped radial sheath. Catheter Cardiovasc Interv 2015;85(1):E35–8.

9. Pancholy SB, Bernat I, Bertrand OF, et al. Prevention of radial artery occlusion after transradial catheterization: the PROPHET-II Randomized Trial. JACC Cardiovasc Interv 2016;9(19):1992–9.

10. Jolly SS, Cairns J, Niemela K, et al. Effect of radial versus femoral access on radiation dose and the importance of procedural volume: a substudy of the multicenter randomized RIVAL trial. JACC Cardiovasc Interv 2013;6(3):258–66.

11. Jolly SS, Yusuf S, Cairns J, et al. Radial versus femoral access for coronary angiography and intervention in patients with acute coronary syndromes (RIVAL): a randomised, parallel group, multicentre trial. Lancet 2011;377(9775):1409–20.

12. Mason PJ, Shah B, Tamis-Holland JE, et al. An update on radial artery access and best practices for transradial coronary angiography and intervention in acute coronary syndrome: a scientific statement from the American Heart Association. Circ Cardiovasc Interv 2018;11(9):e000035.

13. Roffi M, Patrono C, Collet JP, et al. 2015 ESC Guidelines for the management of acute coronary syndromes in patients presenting without persistent ST-segment elevation. Task Force for the Management of Acute Coronary Syndromes in Patients Presenting without Persistent ST-Segment Elevation of the European Society of Cardiology (ESC). G Ital Cardiol 2016;17(10):831–72.

14. Cooper CJ, El-Shiekh RA, Cohen DJ, et al. Effect of transradial access on quality of life and cost of cardiac catheterization: a randomized comparison. Am Heart J 1999;138(3 Pt 1):430–6.

15. Baker NC, O'Connell EW, Htun WW, et al. Safety of coronary angiography and percutaneous coronary intervention via the radial versus femoral route in patients on uninterrupted oral anticoagulation with warfarin. Am Heart J 2014;168(4):537–44.

16. Larsen P, Shah S, Waxman S, et al. Comparison of procedural times, success rates, and safety between left versus right radial arterial access in primary percutaneous coronary intervention for acute ST-segment elevation myocardial infarction. Catheter Cardiovasc Interv 2011;78(1):38–44.

17. Le J, Bangalore S, Guo Y, et al. Predictors of access site crossover in patients who underwent transradial coronary angiography. Am J Cardiol 2015;116(3):379–83.

18. Burzotta F, Trani C, Mazzari MA, et al. Vascular complications and access crossover in 10,676 transradial percutaneous coronary procedures. Am Heart J 2012;163(2):230–8.

19. Valgimigli M, Campo G, Penzo C, et al. Transradial coronary catheterization and intervention across the whole spectrum of Allen test results. J Am Coll Cardiol 2014;63(18):1833–41.

20. Bertrand OF, Carey PC, Gilchrist IC. Allen or no Allen: that is the question! J Am Coll Cardiol 2014;63(18):1842–4.

21. Sciahbasi A, Calabro P, Sarandrea A, et al. Randomized comparison of operator radiation exposure comparing transradial and transfemoral approach for percutaneous coronary procedures: rationale and design of the minimizing adverse haemorrhagic events by TRansradial access site and systemic implementation of angioX - RAdiation Dose study (RAD-MATRIX). Cardiovasc Revasc Med 2014;15(4):209–13.

22. Sciahbasi A, Frigoli E, Sarandrea A, et al. Determinants of radiation dose during right transradial access: insights from the RAD-MATRIX study. Am Heart J 2018;196:113–8.

23. Sciahbasi A, Rigattieri S, Sarandrea A, et al. Operator radiation exposure during right or left transradial coronary angiography: a phantom study. Cardiovasc Revasc Med 2015;16(7):386–90.

24. Shah B, Burdowski J, Guo Y, et al. Effect of Left Versus Right Radial Artery Approach for Coronary Angiography on Radiation Parameters in Patients With Predictors of Transradial Access Failure. Am J Cardiol 2016;118(4):477–81.

25. Tejas Patel SS, Ranjan A. Patel's atlas of transradial intervention: the basics and beyond. 1st edition 2007.

26. Seto AH, Roberts JS, Abu-Fadel MS, et al. Real-time ultrasound guidance facilitates transradial access: RAUST (Radial Artery access with Ultrasound Trial). JACC Cardiovasc Interv 2015;8(2):283–91.

27. Pancholy SB, Sanghvi KA, Patel TM. Radial artery access technique evaluation trial: randomized comparison of Seldinger versus modified Seldinger technique for arterial access for transradial catheterization. Catheter Cardiovasc Interv 2012;80(2):288–91.

28. Bernat I, Abdelaal E, Plourde G, et al. Early and late outcomes after primary percutaneous coronary intervention by radial or femoral approach in patients presenting in acute ST-elevation myocardial infarction and cardiogenic shock. Am Heart J 2013;165(3):338–43.

29. Baumann F, Roberts JS. Evolving techniques to improve radial/ulnar artery access: crossover rate of 0.3% in 1,000 consecutive patients undergoing cardiac catheterization and/or percutaneous coronary intervention via the wrist. J Interv Cardiol 2015;28(4):396–404.

30. Baumann F, Roberts JS. Real time intraprocedural ultrasound measurements of the radial and ulnar arteries in 565 consecutive patients undergoing cardiac catheterization and/or percutaneous coronary intervention via the wrist: understanding anatomy and anomalies may improve access success. J Interv Cardiol 2015;28(6):574–82.

31. Gilchrist IC, Kozak M. Hydrophilic-coated radial sheaths: a leap forward, but watch where you land. JACC Cardiovasc Interv 2010;3(5):484–5.

32. Rathore S, Stables RH, Pauriah M, et al. Impact of length and hydrophilic coating of the introducer sheath on radial artery spasm during transradial coronary intervention: a randomized study. JACC Cardiovasc Interv 2010;3(5):475–83.

33. Izgi C, Feray H. Is radial access and transradial cardiac catheterization feasible without the use of any vasodilator? Int J Angiol 2014;23(1):41–6.

34. Deftereos S, Giannopoulos G, Raisakis K, et al. Moderate procedural sedation and opioid analgesia during transradial coronary interventions to prevent spasm: a prospective randomized study. JACC Cardiovasc Interv 2013;6(3):267–73.

35. Dharma S, Kedev S, Patel T, et al. The predictors of post-procedural arm pain after transradial approach in 1706 patients underwent transradial catheterization. Cardiovasc Revasc Med 2019;20(8):674–7.

36. Dharma S, Kedev S, Patel T, et al. Post-procedural/pre-hemostasis intra-arterial nitroglycerin after transradial catheterization: a gender based analysis. Cardiovasc Revasc Med 2016;17(1):10–4.

37. Dharma S, Shah S, Radadiya R, et al. Nitroglycerin plus diltiazem versus nitroglycerin alone for spasm prophylaxis with transradial approach. J Invasive Cardiol 2012;24(3):122–5.

38. Kwok CS, Rashid M, Fraser D, et al. Intra-arterial vasodilators to prevent radial artery spasm: a systematic review and pooled analysis of clinical studies. Cardiovasc Revasc Med 2015;16(8):484–90.

39. Pancholy SB. Comparison of the effect of intra-arterial versus intravenous heparin on radial artery occlusion after transradial catheterization. Am J Cardiol 2009;104(8):1083–5.

40. Maden O, Kafes H, Balci KG, et al. Relation Between End-Procedural Activated Clotting Time Values and Radial Artery Occlusion Rate With Standard Fixed-Dose Heparin After Transradial Cardiac Catheterization. Am J Cardiol 2016;118(10):1455–9.

41. Rao SV, Tremmel JA, Gilchrist IC, et al. Best practices for transradial angiography and intervention: a consensus statement from the society for cardiovascular angiography and intervention's transradial

working group. Catheter Cardiovasc Interv 2014; 83(2):228–36.

42. Lippe CM, Reineck EA, Kunselman AR, et al. Warfarin: impact on hemostasis after radial catheterization. Catheter Cardiovasc Interv 2015;85(1):82–8.

43. Pancholy S, Coppola J, Patel T, et al. Prevention of radial artery occlusion-patent hemostasis evaluation trial (PROPHET study): a randomized comparison of traditional versus patency documented hemostasis after transradial catheterization. Catheter Cardiovasc Interv 2008;72(3):335–40.

44. Gupta S, Nathan S. Radial artery use and reuse. Preserving radial patency after transradial catheterization procedures. Cardiac Interventions Today 2015.

45. Khuddus M. Improving patient care and post procedure efficiency following transradial access. Cath lab Digest 2017;25(10). Available at: https://www.cathlabdigest.com/article/Improving-Patient-Care-Post-Procedure-Efficiency-Following-Transradial-Access.

46. Seto AH, Rollefson W, Patel MP, et al. Radial haemostasis is facilitated with a potassium ferrate haemostatic patch: the Statseal with TR Band assessment trial (STAT). EuroIntervention 2018; 14(11):e1236–42.

47. Kiemeneij F. Left distal transradial access in the anatomical snuffbox for coronary angiography (ldTRA) and interventions (ldTRI). EuroIntervention 2017;13(7):851–7.

48. Davies RE, Gilchrist IC. Back hand approach to radial access: the snuff box approach. Cardiovasc Revasc Med 2018;19(3 Pt B):324–6.

49. Corcos T. Distal radial access for coronary angiography and percutaneous coronary intervention: a state-of-the-art review. Catheter Cardiovasc Interv 2019;93(4):639–44.

50. Sgueglia GA, Di Giorgio A, Gaspardone A, et al. Anatomic basis and physiological rationale of distal radial artery access for percutaneous coronary and endovascular procedures. JACC Cardiovasc Interv 2018;11(20):2113–9.

51. Aoi S, Htun WW, Freeo S, et al. Distal transradial artery access in the anatomical snuffbox for coronary angiography as an alternative access site for faster hemostasis. Catheter Cardiovasc Interv 2019. [Epub ahead of print].

52. Roghani-Dehkordi F, Hashemifard O, Sadeghi M, et al. Distal accesses in the hand (two novel techniques) for percutaneous coronary angiography and intervention. ARYA Atheroscler 2018;14(2):95–100.

53. Lee JW, Park SW, Son JW, et al. Real-world experience of the left distal transradial approach for coronary angiography and percutaneous coronary intervention: a prospective observational study (LeDRA). EuroIntervention 2018;14(9):e995–1003.

54. Mizuguchi Y, Izumikawa T, Hashimoto S, et al. Efficacy and safety of the distal transradial approach in

coronary angiography and percutaneous coronary intervention: a Japanese multicenter experience. Cardiovasc Interv Ther 2019. [Epub ahead of print].

55. Norimatsu K, Kusumoto T, Yoshimoto K, et al. Importance of measurement of the diameter of the distal radial artery in a distal radial approach from the anatomical snuffbox before coronary catheterization. Heart Vessels 2019;34(10):1615–20.

56. Hahalis G, Tsigkas G, Xanthopoulou I, et al. Transulnar compared with transradial artery approach as a default strategy for coronary procedures: a randomized trial. The transulnar or transradial instead of coronary transfemoral angiographies study (the AURA of ARTEMIS Study). Circ Cardiovasc Interv 2013;6(3):252–61.

57. Gokhroo R, Bisht D, Padmanabhan D, et al. Feasibility of ulnar artery for cardiac catheterization: AJmer ULnar ARtery (AJULAR) catheterization study. Catheter Cardiovasc Interv 2015; 86(1):42–8.

58. Gokhroo R, Kishor K, Ranwa B, et al. Ulnar artery interventions non-inferior to radial approach: AJmer Ulnar ARtery (AJULAR) Intervention Working Group Study Results. J Invasive Cardiol 2016;28(1):1–8.

59. Fernandez R, Zaky F, Ekmejian A, et al. Safety and efficacy of ulnar artery approach for percutaneous cardiac catheterization: systematic review and meta-analysis. Catheter Cardiovasc Interv 2018; 91(7):1273–80.

60. Sattur S, Singh M, Kaluski E. Transulnar access for coronary angiography and percutaneous coronary intervention. J Invasive Cardiol 2014;26(8):404–8.

61. Dahal K, Rijal J, Lee J, et al. Transulnar versus transradial access for coronary angiography or percutaneous coronary intervention: a meta-analysis of randomized controlled trials. Catheter Cardiovasc Interv 2016;87(5):857–65.

62. Khan S. Ulnar access for catheterization and intervention: when and how radial operators should consider transulnar access as an alternative to transfemoral access. Cardiac Interventions Today 2017; 11(5):47–51.

63. Vassilev D, Smilkova D, Gil R. Ulnar artery as access site for cardiac catheterization: anatomical considerations. J Interv Cardiol 2008;21(1):56–60.

64. Sattur S, Singh M, Kaluski E. Trans-ulnar catheterization and coronary interventions: from technique to outcomes. Cardiovasc Revasc Med 2017;18(4): 299–303.

65. Chugh SK, Chugh S, Chugh Y, et al. Feasibility and utility of pre-procedure ultrasound imaging of the arm to facilitate transradial coronary diagnostic and interventional procedures (PRIMAFACIE-TRI). Catheter Cardiovasc Interv 2013;82(1):64–73.

66. Vikas Singh M, Mauricio G, Cohen MD, et al. Crossover from radial to ipsilateral ulnar access: an additional strategy in the Armamentarium of the

"Radialist". Cath Lab Digest 2015;23(4). Available at: https://www.cathlabdigest.com/article/Crossover-Radial-Ipsilateral-Ulnar-Access-Additional-Strategy-Armamentarium-%22Radialist%22.

67. Kern M. You went ulnar when radial was not suitable. Now how do you close the punctures? Cath Lab Digest 2017;25(10). Available at: https://www.

cathlabdigest.com/article/You-Went-Ulnar-When-Radial-was-Not-Suitable-Now-How-Do-You-Close-Punctures.

68. Kedev S, Zafirovska B, Dharma S, et al. Safety and feasibility of transulnar catheterization when ipsilateral radial access is not available. Catheter Cardiovasc Interv 2014;83(1):E51–60.

Coronary Cannulation
Tips for Success in Transradial Angiography and Interventions

Brett M. Milford, DO, Mauricio G. Cohen, MD, FSCAI*

KEYWORDS

- Transradial angiography • Transradial percutaneous coronary intervention
- Cardiac catheterization • Coronary angiography

KEY POINTS

- Transradial access (TRA) is associated with reduced bleeding risk, length of stay, costs and increased patient satisfaction.
- A common reason for TRA failure is a lack of guiding catheter support. Therefore it is important to understand the physics that govern catheter support and manipulation for TRA catheterization.
- Catheter selection and engagement is crucial for obtaining good-quality angiograms and successfully completing percutaneous coronary intervention.
- The maneuvers required for catheter manipulation and coronary engagement differ between transradial and transfemoral arterial access.
- Dexterity in the use of dedicated universal catheters for TRA coronary cannulation can save time, radiation, and contrast.

INTRODUCTION

Transradial artery access (TRA) for coronary angiography and percutaneous coronary intervention (PCI) can provide several advantages over the transfemoral approach (TFA). Potential benefits include a reduced bleeding risk; trend toward a decrease in ischemic end points of death, stroke, or myocardial infarction; reduced length of stay and costs; early ambulation; and improved patient comfort for most patients.[1,2] A survey conducted in 2016 with more than 1000 responses from 91 countries, including the United States, shows that TRA for diagnostic angiography is most frequently done using 5-French (F) catheters (70.4%) with almost two-thirds using a universal catheter (62.9%).[3] If the operator opts out of a universal catheter, then Judkins left (JL) and Judkins right (JR) catheters remain the most popular catheters, regardless of a right or left radial approach.

For PCI, passive support, single-curve catheters, such as extra backup (EBU), are preferred for the left coronary artery (LCA) and the JR for the right coronary artery (RCA).[3]

PRINCIPLES FOR TRANSRADIAL CATHETERIZATION AND INTERVENTION

The general principles of cardiac catheterization remain the same with either TRA or TFA. Because the radial artery is smaller than the femoral artery, TRA requires an adaption of technique compared with TFA. The radial artery diameter ranges from 3.10 mm ± 0.60 mm in men to 2.80 mm ± 0.60 mm in women.[4] Therefore, the use of large-bore catheters is limited with TRA; however, size limitations can be overcome by using sheathless techniques or dedicated radial catheters with larger inner diameter.[5]

Cardiovascular Division, Department of Medicine, Elaine and Sydney Sussman Cardiac Catheterization Laboratory, University of Miami Hospital and Clinics, UHealth Tower, 1400 Northwest 12th Avenue, Suite 864, Miami, FL 33136, USA
* Corresponding author.
E-mail address: mgcohen@med.miami.edu

Intervent Cardiol Clin 9 (2020) 21–31
https://doi.org/10.1016/j.iccl.2019.08.010
2211-7458/20/© 2019 Elsevier Inc. All rights reserved.

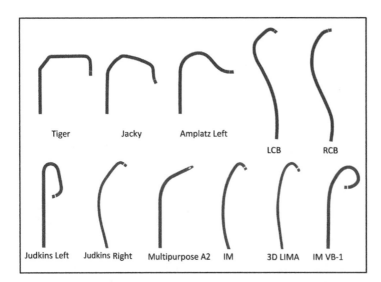

Fig. 1. Most frequently used diagnostic coronary catheter shapes in diagnostic transradial coronary angiography. Multipurpose A2 refers to a slightly longer distal tip than the MP A1. 3D LIMA (Cordis, Santa Clara, California) has a flatter secondary curve than a standard IM catheter. IM, internal mammary; LCB, left coronary bypass; RCB, right coronary bypass.

Some operators have argued that TRA may yield poorer-quality images compared with TFA, in particular for the LCA.[6] Therefore, understanding coronary cannulation technique and catheter selection is critical for obtaining good-quality angiograms with complete opacification of the entire length of the vessel throughout systole and diastole and avoiding noncoaxial engagement. Knowledge of the different catheter shapes is important in order to select the catheter that provides the best backup support and avoids failure. In a large observational study, lack of guiding catheter support because of either extreme subclavian tortuosity or inadequate support was the reason for TRA PCI failure in a third of cases.[7] Fig. 1 displays the most commonly used catheter shapes for transradial coronary angiography. Box 1 includes several practical tips that readers will find useful in their TRA catheterization practice.

> **Box 1**
> **Tips for successful coronary cannulation in transradial catheterization and interventions**
>
> - Use a 260-cm wire with a small J-curve (radius = 1.5 mm) to navigate the upper extremity vasculature.
> - Hydrophilic, stiff, or 0.014-in wires are useful in case of tortuous anatomy.
> - For complex PCI, select catheter shape and size according to coronary anatomy and type of lesion.
> - Always perform catheter exchanges over a wire, with the tip in the aortic root, by either using a 260-cm long or jet exchange with shorter wires.
> - Deep inspiration and turning the head to the left facilitates navigation and straighten tortuosity.
> - Always keep the wire within the guide catheter during manipulations to prevent knotting and kinking.
> - Advance catheter and start manipulation over the wire deep into aortic cusp of interest.
> - Noncoaxial engagement occurs frequently, especially with the LCA. After engagement of the coronary ostium, pull back the catheter gently to improve coaxiality.

DIAGNOSTIC CATHETER SELECTION AND MANIPULATION

Standard femoral catheter shapes, such as the Judkins family of catheters, perform well from the left or right radial approach. Given the trajectory of the catheter when coming from the right subclavian artery, a shorter secondary curve (JL 3.5 instead of JL 4) for the left coronary system is recommended (Fig. 2). The JL catheter is preferred in cases of horizontal aortas with an upward takeoff of the left main coronary artery. To engage the LCA with the JL 3.5 catheter (Fig. 3) the following maneuvers are executed:

- It is advisable to leave the 0.035-in guide wire inside the catheter (but not protruding) to prevent the catheter from folding up during manipulation.
- As the JL catheter is advanced from the innominate artery into the ascending aorta, gentle clockwise torque is applied

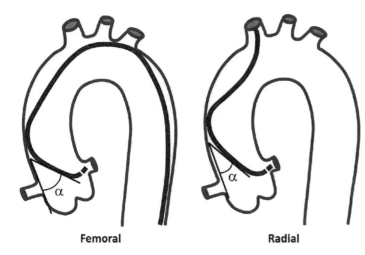

Femoral   **Radial**

Fig. 2. Engagement of the LCA with JL catheters. differences between transradial and transfemoral access. Differential catheter course through transfemoral and transradial vascular access. Because of the curvature between the brachiocephalic trunk and the ascending aorta, a shorter secondary curve, usually by 0.5 cm, is needed for successful cannulation of the LCA with a JL catheter. For TRA, operators should select a JL 3.5 instead of a JL 4.0 catheter.

at the hub of the catheter to make the tip point toward the left coronary cusp.

- As the catheter tip approximates the left coronary ostium, fine torque in movements of either direction usually allows for selective cannulation.
- In cases of the tip falling below the ostium, pushing the catheter gently prolapses the secondary curve of the catheter into the sinus of Valsalva and points the tip up toward the ostium.
- Once engaged, ensure the tip of the catheter is coaxial with the vessel by pulling back the catheter with a gentle clockwise torque. Coaxial engagement is crucial to avoid left main dissections with contrast injection.

To engage the RCA, the JR 4, depicted in **Figs. 4** and **5**, remains the most commonly used catheter for RCA cannulation.[3] Manipulating the catheter to engage the RCA from the radial approach is similar to that of the femoral approach. The JR catheter is advanced into the right coronary cusp and then pulled back gently while applying clockwise torque until the catheter finds the ostium of the RCA. A common pitfall is to begin torqueing the catheter before the slack has been fully removed from the catheter by pulling the catheter back.

A single-catheter or universal catheter approach where 1 catheter is used to engage both coronary arteries can be accomplished with various catheter shapes and has various benefits. By reducing the number of catheter exchanges, there is less radial vasospasm, with improved patient comfort.[8] In addition, less fluoroscopy time is required and, therefore, less radiation exposure is accumulated by using a single-catheter technique.[9] Furthermore, universal catheters are more likely to cannulate anomalous or aberrant coronary arteries. In approximately a third of cases, both coronary ostia cannot be selectively engaged with a universal catheter; then, alternative catheters must be utilized. A recent international survey, including responses from more than 1000 interventional cardiologists, indicated that universal

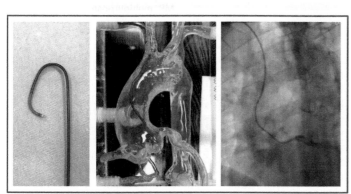

Fig. 3. JL catheter. (*Left*) JL 3.5 guiding catheter. (*Center*) JL 3.5 cannulating the LMCA via R TRA in a 3D printed model of the aortic root, arch and left coronary tree. (*Right*) Fluoroscopic and angiographic appearance of engaging with the JL 3.5.

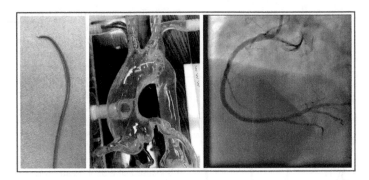

Fig. 4. JR catheter. (*Left*) JR 4 guiding catheter. (*Center*) JR 4 cannulating the RCA via R TRA in a 3D printed model of the aortic root, arch and proximal RCA. (*Right*) Fluoroscopic and angiographic appearance of coaxial engagement, good arterial opacification and adequate reflux of contrast into the aortic root.

catheters are preferred for diagnostic coronary angiography, followed by Judkins catheters, as shown in Fig. 3. Examples of universal catheters include the Kimny (Boston Scientific, Marlborough, Massachusetts), Tiger (Terumo, Tokyo, Japan), Jacky (Terumo), Ultimate (Merit Medical, South Jordan, Utah), DxTerity TRA (Medtronic, Minneapolis, Minnesota), and Ikari (Terumo) catheters. Some universal catheters may also have a side hole just proximal to the tip, which is a safety feature in cases of noncoaxial cannulation. The side hole decompresses a forceful contrast injection and may prevent coronary dissection when the tip of the catheter is directed against the vessel wall. The distal side hole also may allow for nonselective opacification of anomalous or aberrant coronary arteries or allow nonselective opacification of either the left anterior descending artery or circumflex artery in a situation, such as a short left main artery.[10] The Tiger catheter is displayed in Fig. 6. The general technique for engaging the LCA with a universal catheter is similar to engaging with a Judkins catheter.

- LCA engagement
  - Maintain the 0.035-inch J-wire within the catheter.
  - As the catheter advances into the ascending aorta, apply clockwise torqueing and place the tip of the catheter just below the LCA and facing patient left or screen right.
  - Gently and slowly pull back the wire; the catheter tip points upward to engage the left main coronary ostium.
  - A very slight clockwise or counterclockwise rotational torque on the catheter wings assists with coaxial cannulation.
- RCA engagement
  - After LCA angiography is complete, disengage the catheter from the left main by pulling the catheter while applying clockwise torque. This directs the catheter tip to the right side of the ascending aorta.
  - Advance the catheter with a tip slightly pointing right (left in the screen) until it enters the right coronary sinus.
  - Advance the catheter until a small amount of slack is visible in the catheter.
  - Pull back the catheter until the slack is removed.

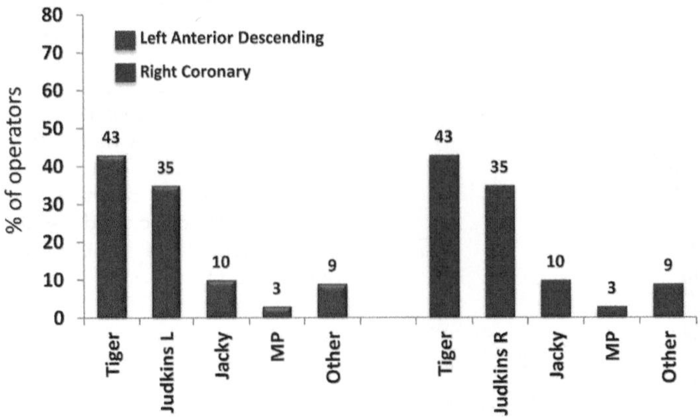

Fig. 5. Catheter preference for diagnostic coronary angiography. MP, multipurpose.

Bar chart showing "% of operators" on the y-axis (0 to 80).

Left Anterior Descending:
- Tiger: 43
- Judkins L: 35
- Jacky: 10
- MP: 3
- Other: 9

Right Coronary:
- Tiger: 43
- Judkins R: 35
- Jacky: 10
- MP: 3
- Other: 9

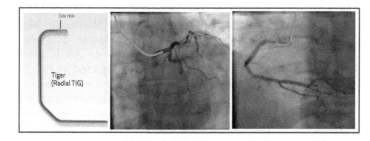

Fig. 6. Universal Tiger catheter for selective cannulation of the right and LCAs. (*Left*) Tiger catheter. (*Center*) shape of Tiger with coaxial engagement of the LMCA. (*Right*) shape of Tiger with coaxial engagement of the RCA. TIG, tiger.

○ Rotate the catheter clockwise until the catheter engages the RCA. A common mistake is clocking the catheter before the catheter slack has been removed. In this situation the tip of the catheter spins 360° after slight pullback.

As soon as the catheter engages a vessel, eyes should go to the arterial pressure. When engaging the RCA, the Tiger catheter, in particular, has a tendency to selectively engage the conus branch. Gently pulling back on the catheter without disengaging and/or a slight counterclockwise rotation can relieve the pressure dampening.

During TRA, torque can build with manipulation and store in the catheter, especially when tortuosity is encountered. This may require a gentle crescendo contrast injection, avoiding a forceful injection, to maintain catheter position. The operator should maintain the right hand on the catheter hub and the left hand on the catheter where it enters the sheath.

The JL 3.5 can selectively engage the RCA by using the stiff back end of a 0.035-in J wire to straighten its secondary curve taking a similar shape to the JR 4. The technique for engaging is similar to a standard JR 4, except that the wire is necessary to straighten the catheter while engaging. When gently engaged, the 0.035-in J wire can be removed and the catheter remains stable.

GUIDE CATHETER SELECTION FOR TRANSRADIAL CORONARY INTERVENTIONS

Equipment for TRA interventions requires a few special considerations. Because of its size, the radial artery can accommodate a guiding catheter of up to 8F as displayed in Table 1, however, a majority of TRA interventions can be

Table 1			
Guiding catheters and device compatibility			
Catheter Diameter	**Type of Device**	**Kissing Balloon**	**Kissing Stents**
5F	Balloon ≤5 mm	No	No
	Stent ≤4.5 mm		
	Intravascular ultrasound		
	PK Papyrus 2.5–4.0 mm		
	Rotational atherectomy (1.25-mm burr)		
6F	All balloon sizes	Yes	No
	All stent sizes		
	Intravascular ultrasound/optical coherence tomography		
	Graftmaster 2.8–4.0 mm//PK Papyrus 4.5–5.0 mm		
	Rotational atherectomy (1.5-mm and 1.75-mm burr)		
	Aspiration thrombectomy catheters		
	Embolic protection devices for SVG interventions		
	Catheter extensions (mother-child/GuideLiner)		
7F	Rotational atherectomy (>1.75 mm burr)	Yes	Yes

Graftmaster covered stent (Abbott, Chicago, IL) Papyrus covered stent (Biotronik, Berlin, Germany)

successfully completed using 5F or 6F guiding catheters. Covered stents, rotational and orbital atherectomy, and/or intravascular ultrasound catheters are compatible with 5F to 6F guide catheters. Even the single-layer PK Papyrus covered stent (Biotronik, Bicester, United Kingdom) can be delivered through 5F or 6F guiding catheters.[11] The advantage of a 5F system versus a 6F system is a smaller arteriotomy, leading to a lower incidence of radial artery occlusion and potentially less vasospasm.[12] Whenever possible, soft tip guides should be selected to avoid catheter-induced arterial injury during engagement or deep-seating maneuvers.

A well-engaged guide with good support is crucial for successful PCI and precise stent delivery. Lack of guide backup support has been reported in up to 17% of cases of failures of TRA PCI.[7] Both active support and passive support of the guiding catheter are important in TRA PCI. With active support, the catheter is manipulated to obtain a stable, coaxial position. TRA may require more careful selection of guiding catheters to increase operational success. **Fig. 7** displays the preferred catheter shapes for right and left coronary interventions.

LEFT CORONARY SYSTEM GUIDING CATHETERS

Most TFA guide shapes are well suited for TRA as well, including the Judkins, Amplatz, and EBU catheters. **Fig. 8** displays some frequently used catheters for the LCA. In TRA PCI, the JL catheters provide less backup support compared with TFA PCI. The angle between the opposite wall of the aorta and the catheter is an important determinant of backup support, with a wider angle associated with greater backup support. JL catheters remain a good option for straightforward interventions of proximal disease and ostial left main coronary lesions. The EBU catheters (EBU [Medtronic, Minneapolis, Minnesota], Voda [Boston Scientific, Marlborough, Massachusetts], or XB [Cordis, Santa Clara, California]), as depicted in **Fig. 9**, offer the most support and are the most widely utilized for the LCA.[3] These catheters provide excellent passive support from the contralateral sinus of Valsalva and allow the catheter to be deep-seated in the sinus. The Ikari left catheters are similar to the JL catheters but have a shorter secondary curve followed by a longer straight distal portion of approximately 20 mm. This straight portion of the Ikari contacts the contralateral aortic wall, which provides backup support and transitions into a tertiary curve. A proximal curve provides support between the innominate artery and the aorta. The available curve sizes include 3.5 (most common), 3.75, and 4.0, which are selected similar to JL sizes. The IL catheter can be used as a universal catheter to engage the left or right coronary systems.[13] The Amplatz left catheters (1 or 2) provide excellent passive backup support and are well suited for complex coronary interventions (ie, calcified lesions and chronic total occlusion).

RIGHT CORONARY SYSTEM GUIDING CATHETERS

Fig. 10 displays the most commonly used catheters for the RCA. The JR guide catheter is the workhorse catheter for a majority of TRA PCIs.[3] A gentle clockwise rotation is applied to the catheter, as from TFA (see **Fig. 10**). The JR 4 may be preferred for ostial lesions and simple RCA lesions. Because the JR 4 does not contact the contralateral aortic wall, it provides little active backup force. Therefore, the JR 4 is not ideal for calcified lesions, tortuous vessels, or

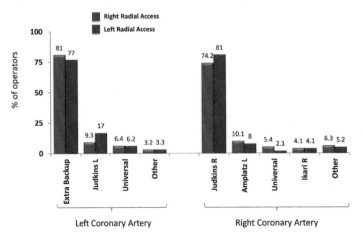

Fig. 7. Guiding catheter preferences for PCI according to right or left radial access.

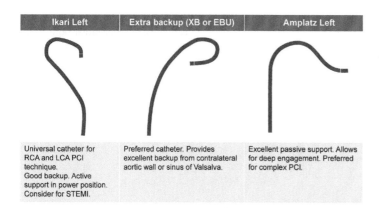

Ikari Left	Extra backup (XB or EBU)	Amplatz Left
Universal catheter for RCA and LCA PCI technique. Good backup. Active support in power position. Consider for STEMI.	Preferred catheter. Provides excellent backup from contralateral aortic wall or sinus of Valsalva.	Excellent passive support. Allows for deep engagement. Preferred for complex PCI.

Fig. 8. Frequently used guiding catheters for transradial left coronary interventions. STEMI, ST elevation myocardial infarction.

chronic occlusions. To improve support, the JR 4 can be deeply intubated into the mid-RCA by applying forward force and clockwise rotation. This maneuver facilitates device delivery and increases backup support but can also cause endothelial injury and vessel dissection. In patients with significantly dilated aortic roots or RCAs that arise anteriorly, the JR 4 does not reach the coronary ostium. The Amplatz right (1 or 2) or Amplatz left (0.75, 1, or 2) may be a better choice and offer adequate backup support. The Amplatz catheter provides additional passive support over the JR, but care must be taken because the Amplatz entails a more aggressive engagement, increasing the risk for catheter-induced traumatic injury to the vessel or aortic wall. The Amplatz catheters engage well into RCAs with a shepherd's crook configuration but are not optimal for very proximal and ostial lesions. Right EBU catheters are the RCA equivalents of left coronary EBU catheters. The Ikari left, EBU, or XB RCA–type curves all provide more backup than JR catheters. The JL

and EBU guides, originally designed for the LCA, also can work well for the RCA. With a 0.035-in guide wire inside the JL or EBU, the catheter takes on a shape similar to a JR or multipurpose, respectively, which makes engagement of the RCA a familiar process for many operators (**Fig. 11**). The JL and EBU, unlike the JR, contacts the contralateral aortic wall, producing greater backup force with increased guide stability during PCI.[14]

Caution must be exercised when engaging and manipulating Amplatz, Ikari left, and active backup support catheters, such as the EBU or XBU catheters. These guide catheters may have a tendency to engage deeply. As a general rule, catheters should be coaxially aligned with the ostium to avoid traumatic iatrogenic dissections. Respiratory variation can cause a back-and-forth motion of the catheter, which can displace the coaxial positioning and lead to a lack of support or traumatic damage to the aorta, ostium, or proximal RCA.

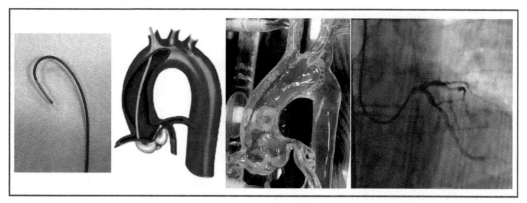

Fig. 9. EBU catheter for transradial left coronary interventions. (*Far left*) EBU guiding catheter. (*Second from left*) Cartoon of EBU showing passive backup support with the secondary curve seated in the right coronary sinus. (*Second from right*) 3D printed model of EBU engaging the LMCA with active support from the contralateral aortic wall. (*Far right*) Fluoroscopic and angiographic appearance of a well-engaged EBU catheter with good active support.

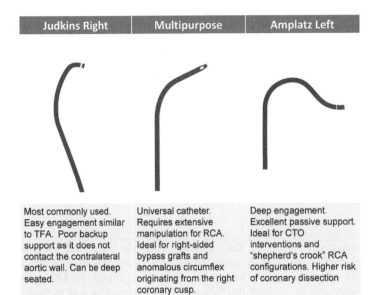

Judkins Right	Multipurpose	Amplatz Left
Most commonly used. Easy engagement similar to TFA. Poor backup support as it does not contact the contralateral aortic wall. Can be deep seated.	Universal catheter. Requires extensive manipulation for RCA. Ideal for right-sided bypass grafts and anomalous circumflex originating from the right coronary cusp.	Deep engagement. Excellent passive support. Ideal for CTO interventions and "shepherd's crook" RCA configurations. Higher risk of coronary dissection

Fig. 10. Frequently used guiding catheters for transradial right coronary interventions.

Other catheters specifically designed for TRA RCA PCI include the Kimny, Ikari right, and Barbeau (Cordis, Santa Clara, California) catheters. These catheters require experience and careful manipulation. The Kimny catheter, for example, has a 45$\underline{o}$ primary curve and a 90$\underline{o}$ secondary curve, which provide contralateral active backup support, and it can be used as a universal catheter for both the left main coronary artery and RCA.[15] The Kimny is engaged from a horizontal or a superior positon and can be helpful for engaging shepherd's crook RCA. The Barbeau catheter is similar to a multipurpose catheter, except the Barbeau has an additional 135$\underline{o}$ curve at the tip. Using the Barbeau, the RCA is cannulated from above the ostium with a clockwise corkscrew maneuver.

SAPHENOUS VEIN GRAFTS

Ascending aortography with approximately 20 mL per second for a total of 40 mL in left anterior oblique can help identify the origin and gross patency of saphenous vein grafts (SVGs). The aortic root angiogram also helps the operator to more optimally select the type of catheter shape required for coaxial

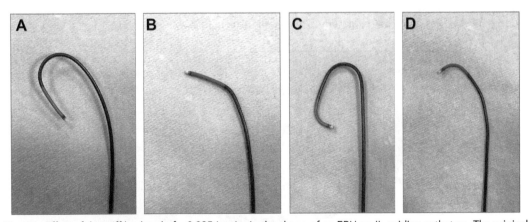

Fig. 11. Effect of the stiff backend of a 0.035-in wire in the shape of an EBU or JL guiding catheters. The original configuration of an EBU catheter (A) can be changed to a multipurpose configuration (B) by straightening the curve with the stiff backend of a 0.035-in wire. Likewise, the original configuration of a JL catheter (C) can be transformed to a JR shape (D). This maneuver facilitates the engagement of the RCA using catheters originally designed for the LCA. Therefore, a multivessel intervention in the left and right coronary arteries can be accomplished without catheter exchanges.

engagement. Accessing SVGs via right radial approach is marginally more challenging than from left radial approach. Although the JR 4 may still engage the left-sided SVGs, the left coronary bypass or Amplatz-type guiding catheters (eg, 1 or 2) are better suited to reach the anterior left and anterior aortic wall. The universal diagnostic catheters may also easily cannulate these left-sided grafts (eg, Tiger or Jacky). For the SVG-RCA/posterior descending artery/posterolateral branch system, the JR 4 generally is a good choice. If the SVG to RCA has a downward, vertical takeoff, a multipurpose catheter may be the guide of choice. In most cases, left TRA results in increased backup support for right-sided grafts compared with right radial access.[16]

INTERNAL MAMMARY ARTERY GRAFTS

The right radial approach is utilized in more than 95% of all TRA cases, but the left radial approach facilitates engagement the left internal mammary artery (LIMA) in patients with a prior history of coronary artery bypass graft surgery.[3] Most operators use a default left TRA strategy for patients with a LIMA bypass. Cannulation of the LIMA is possible, however, via the right radial approach as well.[16,17] Although challenging, the steps to engage the LIMA from the right radial approach include the following:

- A catheter with an angulated primary curve, such as JR 4, is advanced over the wire to the aortic arch.
- The catheter tip is gently turned to point toward the left subclavian artery.
- A soft hydrophilic wire is advanced distally into the axillary/brachial artery.
- The wire is stabilized and fixed by bending the elbow or by inflating a blood pressure cuff on the left arm.
- The catheter initially used to advance the wire into the left subclavian artery is exchanged for a soft 4F internal mammary catheter, which is carefully advanced over the trapped wire without prolapsing into the descending aorta.
- When the catheter reaches the left subclavian artery distal to the origin of the LIMA, the wire is removed and the catheter is withdrawn gently with a gentle counterclockwise torque as the catheter searches for the anterior LIMA ostium. These maneuvers are best performed on 10o of right anterior oblique angiographic view with a slight cranial angulation.

It is obvious that cannulating a LIMA from right radial access requires dexterity with complex catheter manipulations. If the wire comes off the left subclavian during catheter exchanges, the entire maneuver has to be started from the beginning, with additional radiation exposure and catheter manipulations in a potentially atheromatous aortic arch, thereby increasing the risk of embolization stroke.

The right internal mammary artery (RIMA) is a straightforward cannulation from the right radial approach. The RIMA can be challenging, however, because the origin may be perpendicular to the catheter, in which case a VB-1 (Cordis, Santa Clara, California) internal mammary artery catheter with a more acutely angulated tip, similar to a fish hook, allows successful cannulation. An alternative strategy to engage the RIMA is to reshape the catheter tip by bending it and advancing it into the subclavian or innominate artery. If these strategies are not successful, a rail directly into the RIMA can be created by free-wiring the RIMA with a 0.014-in coronary guide wire and tracking a catheter directly to the ostium for angiography.

ANOMALOUS CORONARY ARTERIES AND TRANSRADIAL INTERVENTIONS

Although coronary anomalies and variants are relatively uncommon, a transradial discussion would not be complete without mentioning strategies for successful angiography. There are reports of cases of an anomalous RCA successfully cannulated via TRA after unsuccessful cannulation via TFA.[18] An anterior takeoff of the RCA may require additional catheter length and support, for which the Amplatz left often is the best equipment. The Amplatz left catheter (1, 2, or 3) is also a choice to engage an anomalous RCA arising from the left cusp. The universal (eg, Jacky or Tiger), JL 4, and JL 5 catheters, which have larger secondary curves, also are good options. If these catheters are required, they are pushed deep into the left coronary sinus, which causes the catheter to look anterior and upward, referred to as a U-turn, and prevents cannulation of the LCA and selective engagement of the RCA.[19] The JR 5 and multipurpose catheters are helpful when engaging an anomalous circumflex arising from the right coronary sinus.

IMPROVING PROCEDURAL SUCCESS BY ENHANCING GUIDE CATHETER SUPPORT

Many operators have argued that TRA does not provide the support or allow for the large diameter needed for complex chronic total inclusion (CTO) interventions.[20,21] Therefore, selecting the right catheter shape and size for a particular intervention is crucial to achieve success in TRA PCI. Deep intubation, active backup catheters, mother-child catheter-in-catheter techniques, guide catheter extensions, sheathless catheters, anchoring balloons, and buddy wire techniques are a part of the radial interventionalist's armamentarium.

Soft tip and smaller-diameter guide catheters facilitate deep coronary intubation, although the risk of traumatic injury to the proximal vessel remains, especially if significant disease is present. A larger diameter guide catheter, such as 7F, via TRA may provide more stability and passive backup. Sheathless catheter insertion allows for larger guiding catheter diameters, overcoming the sizing limitations of TRA. There are 2 approaches to sheathless techniques. The first approach includes using a standard 7F to 8F guiding catheter advanced over an 0.035-in wire and a long 125-cm 5F diagnostic catheter that provides a taper and a smooth pass through the arteriotomy and skin.[22] The second approach include the use of dedicated hydrophilic-coated sheathless catheters (Asahi Intecc, Aichi, Japan) with an external diameter of a 6.5F, which is actually smaller than that of a 5F sheath, or 7.5F, smaller than that of a 6F sheath. Therefore, the sheathless system allows large-bore TRA interventions even in patients with small radial arteries. In addition, the hydrophilic coating reduces frictional forces, discomfort, and radial artery spasm.[23] Additional support can be achieved through a buddy wire or a stiffer extra support wire or by placing a second stiff wire in the left anterior descending while intervening in the left circumflex (or vice versa).[24] An anchoring balloon can be placed in a proximal side branch and inflated at low pressure to facilitate advancement of PCI equipment. The mother-child or mother-daughter system can provide additional backup when using 6F catheters and allows for the use of smaller guide catheters to perform deep intubation maneuvers in lesions with severe proximal tortuousity or heavy calcification. A 5-in-6 system, in which a 5F 120-cm long guide catheter is inserted into a 6F 100-cm long guide catheter, also can help provide additional support for delivery of PCI equipment.[25] These techniques have been largely replaced by guide catheter extensions, such as GuideLiner (Teleflex, Morrisville, North Carolina), Guidezilla II (Boston Scientific, Marlborough, Massachusetts), or Telescope (Medtronic, Dublin, Ireland).[26,27] These catheters are the rapid-exchange version of the mother-child system and consist of a 20-cm to 25-cm soft-tipped catheter connected with a metal collar to a 115-cm to 125-cm push wire for advancement and positioning. These guide extensions allow for safer deep intubation of the target vessel, thereby providing additional support when there is difficulty advancing equipment, such as balloons and/or stents across tortuous calcified vessels. Another advantage to the guide-extension catheters is in recanalization of chronic total occlusions, where they can help reestablish a reentry plane in the case of retrograde crossing or reverse controlled anterograde and retrograde subintimal tracking.

FINAL CONSIDERATIONS

TRA coronary angiography and PCI offer significant benefits over TFA. Most coronary procedures can be performed safely and effectively from the transradial approach. Anatomic variants propose special challenges, as they do from the femoral approach, but often these challenges do not prevent successful angiography and subsequent intervention if needed. Guiding catheters should be selected to achieve safe cannulation with optimal support. In general, 6F catheters are adequate for a majority of interventions and 7F thin-walled sheaths and corresponding catheters are available if additional support is required. A sheathless approach can be pursued if an 8F catheter is required. Active backup support catheters should be the preferable equipment for complex anatomy. Although radial specific guide shapes work well, standard-shaped guide catheters work very well and remain common. Universal radial catheters can potentially decrease the duration of the procedure, radiation exposure, and contrast volume and may be ideal for ST elevation myocardial infarction interventions. No one guide catheter has shown superior to others. Guide catheter selection is based on patient anatomy and operator preference. Selecting the optimal guide catheter and careful, correct manipulation remain key to successful TRA coronary angiography and PCI.

REFERENCES

1. Rao SV, Cohen MG, Kandzari DE, et al. The transradial approach to percutaneous coronary intervention: historical perspective, current concepts, and future directions. J Am Coll Cardiol 2010;55(20):2187–95.
2. Bertrand OF, Belisle P, Joyal D, et al. Comparison of transradial and femoral approaches for percutaneous coronary interventions: a systematic review

and hierarchical Bayesian meta-analysis. Am Heart J 2012;163(4):632–48.

3. Shroff AR, Fernandez C, Vidovich MI, et al. Contemporary transradial access practices: Results of the second international survey. Catheter Cardiovasc Interv 2019;93(7):1276–87.

4. Saito S, Ikei H, Hosokawa G, et al. Influence of the ratio between radial artery inner diameter and sheath outer diameter on radial artery flow after transradial coronary intervention. Catheter Cardiovasc Interv 1999;46(2):173–8.

5. Noble S, Tessitore E, Gencer B, et al. A randomized study of sheathless vs standard guiding catheters for transradial percutaneous coronary interventions. Can J Cardiol 2016;32(12):1425–32.

6. Chow WWK, Bing R, Kanawati J, et al. A comparison of image quality using radial vs femoral approaches in patients undergoing diagnostic coronary angiography. J Invasive Cardiol 2018;30(11):411–5.

7. Dehghani P, Mohammad A, Bajaj R, et al. Mechanism and predictors of failed transradial approach for percutaneous coronary interventions. JACC Cardiovasc Interv 2009;2(11):1057–64.

8. Ruiz-Salmeron RJ, Mora R, Velez-Gimon M, et al. Radial artery spasm in transradial cardiac catheterization. Assessment of factors related to its occurrence, and of its consequences during follow-up. Rev Esp Cardiol 2005;58(5):504–11 [in Spanish].

9. Plourde G, Abdelaal E, MacHaalany J, et al. Comparison of radiation exposure during transradial diagnostic coronary angiography with single- or multi-catheters approach. Catheter Cardiovasc Interv 2017;90(2):243–8.

10. De Bruyne B, Stockbroeckx J, Demoor D, et al. Role of side holes in guide catheters: observations on coronary pressure and flow. Cathet Cardiovasc Diagn 1994;33(2):145–52.

11. Kandzari DE, Birkemeyer R. PK Papyrus covered stent: device description and early experience for the treatment of coronary artery perforations. Catheter Cardiovasc Interv, in press.

12. Dahm JB, Vogelgesang D, Hummel A, et al. A randomized trial of 5 vs. 6 French transradial percutaneous coronary interventions. Catheter Cardiovasc Interv 2002;57(2):172–6.

13. Ikari Y, Nagaoka M, Kim JY, et al. The physics of guiding catheters for the left coronary artery in transfemoral and transradial interventions. J Invasive Cardiol 2005;17(12):636–41.

14. Ikari Y, Masuda N, Matsukage T, et al. Backup force of guiding catheters for the right coronary artery in transfemoral and transradial interventions. J Invasive Cardiol 2009;21(11):570–4.

15. Shibata Y, Doi O, Goto T, et al. New guiding catheter for transrad PTCA. Cathet Cardiovasc Diagn 1998;43(3):344–51.

16. Burzotta F, Trani C, Hamon M, et al. Transradial approach for coronary angiography and interventions in patients with coronary bypass grafts: tips and tricks. Catheter Cardiovasc Interv 2008;72(2):263–72.

17. Patel T, Shah S, Patel T. Cannulating LIMA graft using right transradial approach: two simple and innovative techniques. Catheter Cardiovasc Interv 2012;80(2):316–20.

18. Lorin JD, Robin B, Lochow P, et al. The right radial approach for stenting of lesions in the right coronary artery with anomalous take-off from the left sinus of valsalva. J Invasive Cardiol 2000;12(9):478–80.

19. Cohen MG, Tolleson TR, Peter RH, et al. Successful percutaneous coronary intervention with stent implantation in anomalous right coronary arteries arising from the left sinus of valsalva: a report of two cases. Catheter Cardiovasc Interv 2002;55(1):105–8.

20. Alaswad K, Menon RV, Christopoulos G, et al. Transradial approach for coronary chronic total occlusion interventions: Insights from a contemporary multicenter registry. Catheter Cardiovasc Interv 2015;85(7):1123–9.

21. Megaly M, Karatasakis A, Abraham B, et al. Radial versus femoral access in chronic total occlusion percutaneous coronary intervention. circ cardiovasc interv 2019;12(6):e007778.

22. From AM, Gulati R, Prasad A, et al. Sheathless transradial intervention using standard guide catheters. Catheter Cardiovasc Interv 2010;76(7):911–6.

23. Cheaito R, Benamer H, Hovasse T, et al. Feasibility and safety of transradial coronary interventions using a 6.5-F sheathless guiding catheter in patients with small radial arteries. Catheter Cardiovasc Interv 2015;86(1):51–8.

24. Dana A, Barbeau GR. The use of multiple "buddies" during transradial angioplasty in a complex calcified coronary tree. Catheter Cardiovasc Interv 2006;67(3):396–9.

25. Takahashi S, Saito S, Tanaka S, et al. New method to increase a backup support of a 6 French guiding coronary catheter. Catheter Cardiovasc Interv 2004;63(4):452–6.

26. Farooq V, Mamas MA, Fath-Ordoubadi F, et al. The use of a guide catheter extension system as an aid during transradial percutaneous coronary intervention of coronary artery bypass grafts. Catheter Cardiovasc Interv 2011;78(6):847–63.

27. Moynagh A, Garot P, Lefevre T, et al. Angiographic success and successful stent delivery for complex lesions using the GuideLiner five-in-six system- a case report. Am Heart Hosp J 2011;9(1):E44–7.

Transradial Angiography and Intervention in Acute Coronary Syndromes

Elie Akl, MD[a], Mohammed K. Rashid, MD[a],
Ahmad Alshatti, MD[a], Sanjit S. Jolly, MD, MSc[a,b,*]

KEYWORDS

- Transradial angiography • Transradial intervention • Radial artery access
- Acute coronary syndrome

KEY POINTS

- Patients with acute coronary syndromes undergoing angiography and intervention are at an increased risk of bleeding.
- Both access site and non–access site-related bleeding are associated with increased mortality.
- Radial compared with femoral access decreases major bleeding, vascular complications, and major adverse cardiac events in patients with acute coronary syndromes, and may decrease mortality.
- A radial-first strategy should be the default approach in all patients undergoing cardiac catheterization, especially patients with acute coronary syndromes.

INTRODUCTION

Transradial access (TRA) is associated with less bleeding and vascular complications than transfemoral access (TFA) in patients with acute coronary syndromes (ACS).[1,2] A large body of evidence currently supports embracing TRA to improve outcomes in these patients. This is reflected in a 2018 scientific statement from the American Heart Association in which a radial-first approach was strongly recommended in all patients undergoing cardiac catheterization, with a graduated level of center and operator experience for TRA use in patients with ACS.[3]

Bleeding Is an Important Outcome in Patients with Acute Coronary Syndrome

Although advances in adjuvant pharmacotherapy have reduced the risk of ischemic PCI-related complications, the use of antithrombotic agents, especially in the presence of an arteriotomy site, increases the risk of bleeding complications. The incidence of bleeding increases with the acuity of clinical presentation and is higher in patients with ACS compared with those with stable coronary artery disease.[4] Verheugt and colleagues[5] examined the prognostic impact of 30-day bleeding in a combined dataset from the REPLACE 2, ACUITY, and HORIZONS AMI trials that included 17,393 patients with ACS undergoing PCI. The rate of access site bleeding was 2.1% and that of non–access site bleeding was 3.3%. One-year mortality was 2.54% in patients with no bleeding, 6.16% with access site bleeding (relative risk [RR], 2.33; 95% confidence interval [CI], 1.53–3.53), and 14.4% with non–access site bleeding (RR, 5.40; 95% CI, 4.32–6.74). After adjustment, the hazard ratio (HR) of non–access site bleeding was more than double that of access site bleeding (HR, 3.94; 95% CI, 3.07–5.15; $P<.0001$ vs HR, 1.82;

---

[a] Department of Medicine, Division of Cardiology, McMaster University, Room C3-118, DBCVSRI Building, 237 Barton Street East, Hamilton, ON L8L 2X2, Canada; [b] Population Health Research Institute, Hamilton, Ontario, Canada
* Corresponding author. Hamilton General Hospital, Room C3-118, DBCVSRI Building, 237 Barton Street East, Hamilton, Ontario L8L 2X2, Canada.
E-mail address: sanjit.jolly@phri.ca

Intervent Cardiol Clin 9 (2020) 33–40
https://doi.org/10.1016/j.iccl.2019.08.003
2211-7458/20/© 2019 Elsevier Inc. All rights reserved.

95% CI, 1.17–2.83; $P = .008$, respectively), but both were associated with increased mortality. These findings were subsequently corroborated in larger studies.[6,7]

It is unclear whether bleeding is a marker of risk or causal for mortality. Nonetheless, several mechanisms by which bleeding may affect mortality have been proposed. These include premature cessation of dual antiplatelet therapy, blood transfusion-related adverse affects, exaggeration of inflammatory responses, and generation of a prothrombotic milieu through activation of the coagulation cascade.[8] Anemia itself decreases oxygen delivery, increases oxygen demand, and can lead to ischemic events owing to supply–demand mismatch. Regardless of the mechanisms involved, if bleeding increases mortality, then avoiding it should decrease mortality. Multiple strategies can be used to minimize bleeding risk in patients with ACS. Pharmacologic therapies that reduce bleeding in ACS have been associated with reductions in mortality (bivalirudin in HORIZONS AMI[9] and fondaparinux in the OASIS 5 and 6 trials[10]). This finding supports the mechanism that reducing bleeding can lead to reductions in mortality.

RANDOMIZED CONTROLLED TRIALS OF TRANSRADIAL ACCESS VERSUS THE FEMORAL APPROACH IN PATIENTS WITH ACUTE CORONARY SYNDROME

Several large randomized trials comparing the radial versus the femoral approach in the ACS population were published over the past decade. The RadIal vs femorAL access for coronary intervention (RIVAL)[1] trial randomized a total of 7021 patients with ACS with or without ST-segment elevation. The primary outcome of death, myocardial infarction (MI), stroke, or noncoronary artery bypass grafting (CABG) bleeding at 30 days occurred in 3.7% in the TRA group versus 4.0% in the TFA group (HR, 0.92; 95% CI, 0.72–1.17; $P = .50$). The rate of major adverse cardiac events (MACE; composite of death, MI, and stroke) was also similar between the 2 groups (3.2% vs 3.2%; HR, 0.98; 95% CI, 0.76–1.28; $P = .90$). However, many notable findings should be underlined. First, in centers with the highest radial PCI volumes, there was a benefit with TRA over TFA for MACE, major vascular complications, and access site crossover. Second, there was a significant benefit with TRA in patients with ST-segment elevation MI (STEMI). This is detailed in a subsequent section. Third, although major bleeding

did not differ as per the trial-specific definition, a post hoc analysis showed a significant reduction with radial access when the ACUITY trial bleeding definition was used ($P<.0001$). Fourth, the rate of major vascular complications was significantly lower with the radial approach (1.4% vs 3.7%; HR, 0.37; 95% CI, 0.27–0.52; $P<.0001$). This was driven by a reduction in large hematoma and pseudoaneurysm needing closure.

The Minimizing Adverse Haemorrhagic Events by TRansradial Access Site and Systemic Implementation of AngioX (MATRIX) was a large trial of more than 8400 patients with ACS.[2] The primary outcome of MACE was lower with TRA compared with TFA (8.8% vs 10.3%; RR, 0.85; 95% CI, 0.74–0.99; $P = .0307$). Similarly, the second coprimary outcome of a net adverse clinical events (NACE) was also reduced with the radial approach (9.8% vs 11.7%; RR, 0.83; 95% CI, 0.73–0.96; $P = .0092$). The difference was mainly driven by bleeding academic research consortium (BARC) major bleeding unrelated to CABG (1.6% vs 2.3%, RR, 0.67; 95% CI, 0.49–0.92; $P = .0128$) and all-cause mortality (1.6% vs 2.2%; RR, 0.72; 95% CI, 0.53–0.99; $P = .045$).

Transradial Access Versus Transfemoral Access in Patients with an ST Elevation Myocardial Infarction

In the RIVAL-STEMI subgroup of 1958 patients, MACE (HR, 0.59; 95% CI, 0.36–0.95; $P = .031$), NACE (HR, 0.60; 95% CI, 0.38–0.94, $P = .026$), and all-cause mortality (HR, 0.39; 95% CI, 0.20–0.76; $P = .006$) were decreased with radial access.[11] ACUITY major bleeding (HR, 0.49; 95% CI, 0.28–0.84; $P = .009$) and major vascular access site complications (HR, 0.36; 95% CI, 0.19–0.70; $P = .002$) were also significantly lower in the radial group. Another subgroup analysis of the 1451 patients treated with primary PCI showed a mortality benefit with TRA (HR, 0.46; 95% CI, 0.22–0.97; $P = .041$).

TRA provided consistent benefits in patients with NSTE-ACS and STEMI at presentation in a prespecified subanalysis of the MATRIX trial.[12] Access site BARC 2 to 5 bleeding was significantly reduced in the radial group irrespective of ACS presentation, as well.

The Radial vs Femoral Randomized Investigation in ST-Elevation Acute Coronary Syndrome (RIFLE-STEACS) trial randomized 1001 patients with STEMI undergoing primary or rescue (8%) PCI to TRA or TFA.[13] The composite primary outcome of death, MI, stroke, target lesion revascularization, or non-CABG bleeding at 30 days was significantly lower in the TRA arm

(13.6% vs 21%; 95% CI, 2.7%–12.0%; P = .003). There was also a significant reduction in cardiac mortality (5.2% vs 9.2%; 95% CI, 0.8%–7.3%; P = .020). Non–CABG-related bleeding was significantly reduced with TRA (7.8% vs 12.2%, 95% CI, 2.7–12.0; P = .026), mainly owing to a 60% decrease in access site-related bleeding (2.6% vs 6.8%; 95% CI, 1.6%–7.0%; P = .002).

The ST Elevation Myocardial Infarction Treated by RADIAL or femoral approach (STEMI-RADIAL) trial included 707 patients undergoing primary PCI by high-volume operators experienced in both access sites.[14] The composite primary end point of major bleeding and vascular access site complications at 30 days was lower with TRA (1.4% vs 7.2%; P = .0001). The NACE rate was also reduced with the radial approach (4.6% vs 11.0%; P = .0028). There was a nonsignificant 26% relative reduction in mortality at 30 days and 36% at 6 months with TRA.

In the most recent trial, Safety and Efficacy of Femoral Access vs Radial Access in ST-Elevation Myocardial Infarction (SAFARI-STEMI), the primary outcome of death at 30 days (1.5% vs 1.3%; RR, 1.15; 95% CI, 0.58–2.30; P = .69), MACE (4% vs 3.4%; RR, 1.17; 95% CI, 0.77–1.79; P = .45), and major bleeding (1.1% vs 1.3%; P = .74) were all not different among the 2 groups. However, the trial was stopped early, having recruited only 2292 of the original target of 4884 patients. As a result, it is likely that SAFARI did not have sufficient power to test the hypothesis, which makes it difficult to draw any firm conclusion. The totality of the data shows that radial improves outcomes compared with femoral access in STEMI.

Meta-analysis of Randomized Trials

An updated meta-analysis of randomized trials of TRA versus TFA in ACS with clinical outcomes available at 30 days demonstrates a trend favoring TRA for MACE, defined as death from any cause (or cardiac death when all-cause mortality was not available), MI or stroke (odds ratio [OR], 0.86; 95% CI, 0.72–1.02; P = .08; I^2 = 6%) (Fig. 1).[11–17] Radial access was associated with a decreased risk of 30-day mortality (OR, 0.71; 95% CI, 0.56–0.90; P = .004; I^2 = 0%), major bleeding (OR, 0.55; 95% CI, 0.41–0.73; P<.0001; I^2 = 24%), and vascular access complications (OR, 0.32; 95% CI, 0.20–0.52; P<.00001; I^2 = 0%) at 30 days. Our findings are highly consistent with prior meta-analyses.[18–22]

The evidence overwhelmingly supports a radial first approach and this is reflected in guidelines from the American Heart Association,

the Canadian Cardiovascular Society/Canadian Association of Intervention Cardiology, and the European Society of Cardiology/European Association for Cardio-Thoracic Surgery, which have all endorsed the radial approach as the preferred site for PCI[3,23,24] (Table 1).

There has previously been concerns that TRA might prolong door-to-balloon times, but contemporary studies of TRA versus TFA failed to demonstrate a significant difference in these times.[1,4,13,25] Furthermore, sensitivity analysis using the mortality benefit seen in large randomized controlled trials with TRA suggests that the small increment in door-to-balloon times is unlikely to affect clinical benefit.[26]

Although radial adoption in the United States has been not as rapid as Europe and Canada, the use of the transradial approach is growing steadily. Data from the American College of Cardiology National Cardiovascular data registry has documented a greater than 6-fold increase of the radial access in primary PCI between 2007 and 2011.[27] Although encouraging, these rates remain much lower than those reported in European countries such as Sweden and the UK, which increased from 10% to 12.5% to 55% to 60% during the same period.[28,29] These numbers underline the need for continuing education for TRA.

TRANSRADIAL ACCESS IN RESCUE PERCUTANEOUS CORONARY INTERVENTION

Bleeding complications in with patients with STEMI who receive fibrinolysis and undergo rescue PCI are relatively common. Thus, determining the optimal access approach for these patients is of particular interest.

In the RADIAL-AMI pilot randomized trial, 50 patients requiring either primary (one-third) or rescue PCI (two-thirds) were randomized to radial versus femoral access. There was a trend toward less hematoma and less hemoglobin decrease (>30 g/L) in the radial group.[15] Data from the Scottish Coronary Revascularisation Register that included 4534 patients undergoing primary or rescue PCI between 2000 and 2009 showed a striking reduction in 30-day mortality (adjusted OR. 0.51; 95% CI, 0.04–0.52; P<.001), greater procedural success, and less access site complications or bleeding with the radial approach.[30] The largest evaluation of outcomes after rescue PCI via TRA versus TFA is from the American College of Cardiology National Cardiovascular Data

A

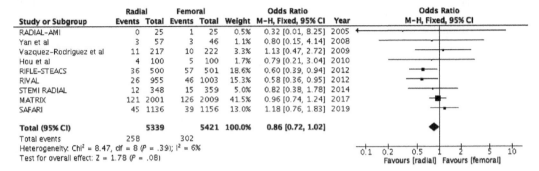

B

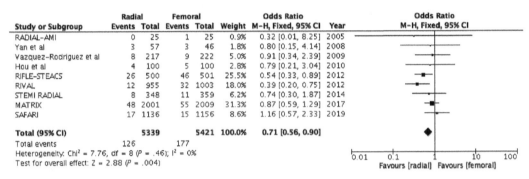

C

Study or Subgroup	Radial Events	Radial Total	Femoral Events	Femoral Total	Weight	Odds Ratio M-H, Fixed, 95% CI	Year
RADIAL-AMI	0	25	0	25		Not estimable	2005
Yan et al	0	57	1	46	1.3%	0.26 [0.01, 6.63]	2008
Vazquez-Rodriguez et al	1	217	5	222	3.8%	0.20 [0.02, 1.73]	2009
Hou et al	0	100	3	100	2.7%	0.14 [0.01, 2.72]	2010
RIFLE-STEACS	9	500	14	501	10.6%	0.64 [0.27, 1.49]	2012
RIVAL	8	955	9	1003	6.7%	0.93 [0.36, 2.43]	2012
STEMI RADIAL	5	348	26	359	19.5%	0.19 [0.07, 0.49]	2014
MATRIX	36	2001	58	2009	44.0%	0.62 [0.40, 0.94]	2017
SAFARI	12	1136	15	1156	11.4%	0.81 [0.38, 1.74]	2019
Total (95% CI)		**5339**		**5421**	**100.0%**	**0.55 [0.41, 0.73]**	
Total events	71		131				

Heterogeneity: Chi² = 9.25, df = 7 (P = .24); I² = 24%
Test for overall effect: Z = 4.10 (P<.0001)

Favours [radial]   Favours [femoral]

Fig. 1. Forest plots of pooled estimates of (A) MACE, (B) death, (C) major bleeding, (D) stroke, and (E) vascular access complications. MACE, major adverse cardiovascular events, defined as the composite of death, MI, and stroke.

Registry.[31] In total, 9494 patients undergoing rescue PCI between 2009 and 2013 were studied. Coronary angiography was performed at a median time of 189 minutes after fibrinolytic therapy. Only 14.2% of cases were performed transradially. Rescue PCI success rates were high and not different between groups (96.1% radial vs 94.7% femoral; P = .06). In propensity-matched analyses, transradial rescue PCI was associated with lower bleeding rates compared with the transfemoral approach (OR, 0.67; 95% CI, 0.52–0.97; P = .003), but not

mortality (OR, 0.81; 95% CI, 0.53–1.25; P = .35). The very low in-hospital mortality (1%–2%) observed in this patient group as compared with data from all-comers with STEMI (in-hospital mortality, 5.5%)[32] could potentially explain the inability to demonstrate a mortality difference with TRA.

Given the proven decrease in bleeding end points with TRA, one should expect an incremental benefit with radial access in patients at highest risk of bleeding, including patients with STEMI undergoing rescue PCI.

D

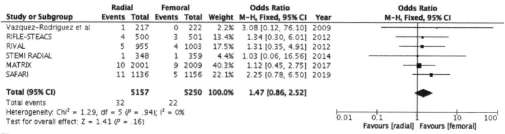

Study or Subgroup	Radial Events	Total	Femoral Events	Total	Weight	Odds Ratio M-H, Fixed, 95% CI	Year
Vazquez-Rodriguez et al	1	217	0	222	2.2%	3.08 [0.12, 76.10]	2009
RIFLE-STEACS	4	500	3	501	13.4%	1.34 [0.30, 6.01]	2012
RIVAL	5	955	4	1003	17.5%	1.31 [0.35, 4.91]	2012
STEMI RADIAL	1	348	1	359	4.4%	1.03 [0.06, 16.56]	2014
MATRIX	10	2001	9	2009	40.3%	1.12 [0.45, 2.75]	2017
SAFARI	11	1136	5	1156	22.1%	2.25 [0.78, 6.50]	2019
Total (95% CI)		**5157**		**5250**	**100.0%**	**1.47 [0.86, 2.52]**	
Total events	32		22				

Heterogeneity: Chi² = 1.29, df = 5 (P = .94); I² = 0%
Test for overall effect: Z = 1.41 (P = .16)

E

Study or Subgroup	Radial Events	Total	Femoral Events	Total	Weight	Odds Ratio M-H, Fixed, 95% CI	Year
RADIAL-AMI	2	25	7	25	9.2%	0.22 [0.04, 1.21]	2005
Yan et al	1	57	6	46	9.3%	0.12 [0.01, 1.03]	2008
Hou et al	3	100	8	100	11.0%	0.36 [0.09, 1.38]	2010
RIFLE-STEACS	1	500	2	501	2.8%	0.50 [0.05, 5.53]	2012
RIVAL	12	955	35	1003	47.9%	0.35 [0.18, 0.68]	2012
STEMI RADIAL	1	348	3	359	4.2%	0.34 [0.04, 3.30]	2014
MATRIX	4	2001	11	2009	15.6%	0.36 [0.12, 1.14]	2017
Total (95% CI)		**3986**		**4043**	**100.0%**	**0.32 [0.20, 0.52]**	
Total events	24		72				

Heterogeneity: Chi² = 1.26, df = 6 (P = .97); I² = 0%
Test for overall effect: Z = 4.71 (P<.00001)

Fig. 1. (*continued*)

TRANSRADIAL ACCESS IN FEMALE PATIENTS WITH ACUTE CORONARY SYNDROME

Female patients with ACS are more likely than males to suffer from bleeding and vascular complications.[33,34] Concerns that TRA might be more challenging in females owing to smaller radial arteries that may be more prone to spasm make sex-specific data regarding the efficacy and safety of TRA very pertinent.

Sex-based outcomes in ACS randomized to TRA versus TFA were compared in a prespecified RIVAL subgroup analysis.[33] Bleeding and major vascular complications were significantly reduced with TRA in both sexes. However, the number needed to treat to prevent 1 major vascular complication was 33 in females compared with 49 for males. Crossover rates were higher with TRA compared with TFA in both women and men, but more so in women (women: 11.1% vs 1.9%; HR. 5.88; P<.0001; men: 6.3% vs 1.9%; HR, 3.32; P<.0001). PCI success rate did not differ by sex, irrespective of access site (female: HR, 1.05, P = .471; male: HR, 1.0; P = .888; P_{int} = .674). When asked about their access preference for a hypothetical repeat procedure, 86.1% of females with TRA preferred TRA, whereas only 50.1% of females with TFA preferred TFA (P<.001).

In an analysis of the MATRIX trial,[34] when comparing TRA versus TFA between females and males with ACS, major adverse cardiovascular and cerebrovascular events, and NACE were significantly lower with TRA in females (major adverse cardiovascular and cerebrovascular events: 9.1% vs 12.2%; RR, 0.73; 95% CI, 0.56–0.95; P = .019; NACE: 10.4% vs 13.9%; RR, 0.73; 95% CI, 0.56–0.93; P = .012), but these reductions only trended favorably for radial in

Table 1
International Society guidelines for radial access in primary PCI

Society	Year	TRA in Primary PCI
CCS – STEMI Guidelines[23]	2019	Strong recommendation, moderate-quality evidence
AHA – Scientific Statement[3]	2018	Strong recommendation
ESC/EACTS Guidelines on Myocardial Revascularization[24]	2018	Class I indication

Abbreviations: AHA, American Heart Association; CCS, Canadian Cardiovascular Society; EACTS, European Association for cardio-thoracic surgery; ESC, European Society of cardiology.

Table 2
TRA versus TFA in females versus males

	TRA vs TFA in Females	TRA vs TFA in Males
Vascular complications	↓↓	↓
Bleeding	↓↓	↓
Crossover	↑↑	↑
PCI success	=	=
MACE	↓	↓/=

Abbreviation: MACCE, major adverse cardiovascular and cerebrovascular event.

males. BARC type 3 or 5 bleeding (P_{int} = .45) and all-cause mortality (P_{int} = 0.79) were lower with TRA in both sexes.

SAFE-PCI for Women is the first randomized trial of PCI strategies performed solely in women. It differs from the above-mentioned studies in that it focused on elective referrals for angiography and PCI, and excluded patients with STEMI.[35] A total of 1787 female patients were randomized to TRA versus TFA, with 691 undergoing PCI. Unfortunately, the trial was stopped prematurely owing to a lower than expected event rate. There was a significant reduction in bleeding and vascular complications with TRA in the overall population (0.6% vs 1.7%; OR, 0.32; 95% CI, 0.12–0.90). There was only a trend toward benefit in the PCI group, most likely owing to the small sample size. Crossover rates were significantly higher with TRA compared with TFA (6.7% vs 1.9%; OR, 3.70; 95% CI, 2.14–6.40). Compared with women assigned to TFA, more women assigned to TRA preferred the same access route for their next procedure (71.9% vs 23.5%).

TRA is effective at significantly reducing bleeding, major vascular complications and MACE in women with similar PCI success rates compared with TFA (Table 2). The radial-first approach is especially applicable to female patients who are at increased baseline risk of bleeding and vascular complications. Continuous efforts should be made to overcome the technical challenges with TRA in females, including gaining expertise in the use of 4F or 5F catheters to minimize the risk of spasm.

SUMMARY

Considerable evidence supports TRA for angiography and intervention in patients with ACS, with an emphasis on decreasing major bleeding and access site vascular complications. Patients undergoing invasive treatment for ACS are at greatest risk of bleeding and have the most to gain. The benefits of TRA have been demonstrated across the ACS spectrum and in both sexes. A radial-first strategy should be the default approach in the ACS population and continuous efforts should be made to increase operator expertise of TRA in these patients.

REFERENCES

1. Jolly SS, Yusuf S, Cairns J, et al. Radial versus femoral access for coronary angiography and intervention in patients with acute coronary syndromes (RIVAL): a randomised, parallel group, multicentre trial. Lancet 2011;377(9775):1409–20.
2. Valgimigli M, Gagnor A, Calabro P, et al. Radial versus femoral access in patients with acute coronary syndromes undergoing invasive management: a randomised multicentre trial. Lancet 2015; 385(9986):2465–76.
3. Mason PJ, Shah B, Tamis-Holland JE, et al. An update on radial artery access and best practices for transradial coronary angiography and intervention in acute coronary syndrome: a scientific statement from the American Heart Association. Circ Cardiovasc Interv 2018;11(9):e000035.
4. Rao SV, Cohen MG, Kandzari DE, et al. The transradial approach to percutaneous coronary intervention: historical perspective, current concepts, and future directions. J Am Coll Cardiol 2010;55(20): 2187–95.
5. Verheugt FW, Steinhubl SR, Hamon M, et al. Incidence, prognostic impact, and influence of antithrombotic therapy on access and nonaccess site bleeding in percutaneous coronary intervention. JACC Cardiovasc Interv 2011;4(2):191–7.
6. Kwok Chun S, Khan Muhammad A, Rao Sunil V, et al. Access and non–access site bleeding after percutaneous coronary intervention and risk of subsequent mortality and major adverse cardiovascular events. Circ Cardiovasc Interv 2015;8(4): e001645.
7. Chhatriwalla AK, Amin AP, Kennedy KF, et al. Association between bleeding events and in-hospital mortality after percutaneous coronary intervention bleeding events and mortality after PCI. JAMA 2013;309(10):1022–9.
8. Bassand JP. Impact of anaemia, bleeding, and transfusions in acute coronary syndromes: a shift in the paradigm. Eur Heart J 2007;28(11):1273–4.
9. Stone GW, Witzenbichler B, Guagliumi G, et al. Bivalirudin during primary PCI in acute myocardial infarction. N Engl J Med 2008;358(21):2218–30.

10. Fifth Organization to Assess Strategies in Acute Ischemic Syndromes Investigators, Yusuf S, Mehta SR, Chrolavicius S, et al. Comparison of fondaparinux and enoxaparin in acute coronary syndromes. N Engl J Med 2006;354(14):1464–76.

11. Mehta SR, Jolly SS, Cairns J, et al. Effects of radial versus femoral artery access in patients with acute coronary syndromes with or without ST-segment elevation. J Am Coll Cardiol 2012; 60(24):2490–9.

12. Vranckx P, Frigoli E, Rothenbuhler M, et al. Radial versus femoral access in patients with acute coronary syndromes with or without ST-segment elevation. Eur Heart J 2017;38(14):1069–80.

13. Romagnoli E, Biondi-Zoccai G, Sciahbasi A, et al. Radial versus femoral randomized investigation in ST-segment elevation acute coronary syndrome: the RIFLE-STEACS (Radial Versus Femoral Randomized Investigation in ST-Elevation Acute Coronary Syndrome) study. J Am Coll Cardiol 2012; 60(24):2481–9.

14. Bernat I, Horak D, Stasek J, et al. ST-segment elevation myocardial infarction treated by radial or femoral approach in a multicenter randomized clinical trial: the STEMI-RADIAL trial. J Am Coll Cardiol 2014;63(10):964–72.

15. Cantor WJ, Puley G, Natarajan MK, et al. Radial versus femoral access for emergent percutaneous coronary intervention with adjunct glycoprotein IIb/IIIa inhibition in acute myocardial infarction–the RADIAL-AMI pilot randomized trial. Am Heart J 2005;150(3):543–9.

16. Yan ZX, Zhou YJ, Zhao YX, et al. Safety and feasibility of transradial approach for primary percutaneous coronary intervention in elderly patients with acute myocardial infarction. Chin Med J (Engl) 2008;121(9):782–6.

17. Hou L, Wei YD, Li WM, et al. Comparative study on transradial versus transfemoral approach for primary percutaneous coronary intervention in Chinese patients with acute myocardial infarction. Saudi Med J 2010;31(2):158–62.

18. Nardin M, Verdoia M, Barbieri L, et al. Radial vs femoral approach in acute coronary syndromes: a meta- analysis of randomized trials. Curr Vasc Pharmacol 2017;16(1):79–92.

19. Bavishi C, Panwar SR, Dangas GD, et al. Meta-analysis of radial versus femoral access for percutaneous coronary interventions in non-ST-segment elevation acute coronary syndrome. Am J Cardiol 2016;117(2):172–8.

20. Khan SA, Harper Y, Slomka T, et al. An updated comprehensive meta-analysis of randomized controlled trials comparing radial versus femoral access for percutaneous interventions in patients with acute coronary syndrome. J Am Coll Cardiol 2016;67(13 Supplement):89.

21. Ferrante G, Rao SV, Juni P, et al. Radial versus femoral access for coronary interventions across the entire spectrum of patients with coronary artery disease: a meta-analysis of randomized trials. JACC Cardiovasc Interv 2016;9(14):1419–34.

22. Ando G, Capodanno D. Radial access reduces mortality in patients with acute coronary syndromes: results from an updated trial sequential analysis of randomized trials. JACC Cardiovasc Interv 2016; 9(7):660–70.

23. Wong GC, Welsford M, Ainsworth C, et al. 2019 Canadian Cardiovascular Society/Canadian Association of Interventional Cardiology guidelines on the acute management of ST-elevation myocardial infarction: focused update on regionalization and reperfusion. Can J Cardiol 2019;35(2):107–32.

24. Neumann FJ, Sousa-Uva M, Ahlsson A, et al. 2018 ESC/EACTS guidelines on myocardial revascularization. Eur Heart J 2019;40(2):87–165.

25. Ratib K, Mamas MA, Anderson SG, et al. Access site practice and procedural outcomes in relation to clinical presentation in 439,947 patients undergoing percutaneous coronary intervention in the United kingdom. JACC Cardiovasc Interv 2015;8(1 Pt A):20–9.

26. Wimmer NJ, Cohen DJ, Wasfy JH, et al. Delay in reperfusion with transradial percutaneous coronary intervention for ST-elevation myocardial infarction: might some delays be acceptable? Am Heart J 2014;168(1):103–9.

27. Baklanov DV, Kaltenbach LA, Marso SP, et al. The prevalence and outcomes of transradial percutaneous coronary intervention for ST-segment elevation myocardial infarction: analysis from the National Cardiovascular Data Registry (2007 to 2011). J Am Coll Cardiol 2013;61(4):420–6.

28. Ratib K, Mamas M, Large A, et al. TCT-26 radial vs femoral access for primary PCI, observational data from the British Cardiovascular Intervention Society Database. J Am Coll Cardiol 2012;60(17 Supplement):B8.

29. SCAAR Annual Report 2011. Scand Cardiovasc J 2013;47(Suppl 62):55–76.

30. Johnman C, Pell JP, Mackay DF, et al. Clinical outcomes following radial versus femoral artery access in primary or rescue percutaneous coronary intervention in Scotland: retrospective cohort study of 4534 patients. Heart 2012;98(7):552–7.

31. Kadakia MB, Rao SV, McCoy L, et al. Transradial versus transfemoral access in patients undergoing rescue percutaneous coronary intervention after fibrinolytic therapy. JACC Cardiovasc Interv 2015; 8(14):1868–76.

32. Roe MT, Messenger JC, Weintraub WS, et al. Treatments, trends, and outcomes of acute myocardial infarction and percutaneous coronary intervention. J Am Coll Cardiol 2010;56(4):254–63.

33. Pandie S, Mehta SR, Cantor WJ, et al. Radial versus femoral access for coronary angiography/intervention in women with acute coronary syndromes: insights from the RIVAL Trial (Radial Vs femorAL access for coronary intervention). JACC Cardiovasc Interv 2015;8(4):505–12.

34. Gargiulo G, Ariotti S, Vranckx P, et al. Impact of sex on comparative outcomes of radial versus femoral access in patients with acute coronary syndromes undergoing invasive management: data from the randomized MATRIX-access trial. JACC Cardiovasc Interv 2018;11(1):36–50.

35. Rao SV, Hess CN, Barham B, et al. A registry-based randomized trial comparing radial and femoral approaches in women undergoing percutaneous coronary intervention: the SAFE-PCI for Women (Study of Access Site for Enhancement of PCI for Women) trial. JACC Cardiovasc Interv 2014;7(8):857–67.

RadialFirst in CHIP and Cardiogenic Shock

Rhian E. Davies, DO, MS, Kathleen E. Kearney, MD, James M. McCabe, MD*

KEYWORDS

- Transradial arterial access • Cardiogenic shock • Alternative access • Large bore access
- Ultrasound guidance access • Antecubital vein

KEY POINTS

- Transradial arterial access is safe and effective for performing high-risk percutaneous coronary interventions, including heavily calcified lesions, bifurcations, and chronic total occlusions.
- Transradial arterial access has improved outcomes, including decreased bleeding and vascular complications.
- Ultrasound can provide information regarding the course of the radial artery and highlight areas of concern.
- The antecubital vein is a viable option into the venous system.
- Axillary arterial access offers advantages for large bore access when required for hemodynamic support in cardiogenic shock or other invasive procedures. In addition, this access site allows quicker ambulation and increased patient comfort.

INTRODUCTION

With the development of smaller sheaths and catheter sizes, as well as favorable hard outcomes data, upper extremity vascular access is an increasingly popular choice by interventionalists. The access site is being used not only for diagnostic cardiac catheterizations but also for hemodynamic assessment, placement of support devices, and subsequent percutaneous coronary interventions (PCI). Growing use of the transradial arterial (TRA) access has resulted in significant reduction of complications. A recent meta-analysis by Ferrante and colleagues[1] evaluating TRA access included 22,843 patients across the spectrum of coronary artery disease (acute coronary syndromes [ACS] and stable ischemic heart disease) requiring coronary angiography and PCI and found 3 main outcomes. First, the use of TRA access compared with transfemoral arterial (TFA) access is associated with a significant 29% relative risk reduction in all-cause mortality and a 16% relative risk reduction in major adverse cardiovascular events (MACE). Second, TRA access was associated with a lower risk for major bleeding and major vascular complications (reduced by 47% and 77%, respectively).[1] Lastly, the rates of myocardial infarction (MI) and stroke after TRA access intervention were comparable with those of TFA access.[1] These findings were similar to a recent publication by Jolly and colleagues[2] who reported decreased vascular complications with subsequent decreased bleeding risk. TRA, if performed by an experienced interventionalist, is now the recommended access site by the 2018 European Society of Cardiology (ESC/EACTS) guidelines for patients with STEMI[3] and in patients with ACS per the 2018 American Heart Association scientific statement.[4]

Despite this evidence and guideline support, a risk–treatment paradox exists for the use of TRA access.[5] Even after excluding patients on hemodialysis and patients who require the use of hemodynamic support, the patients who are

---

Disclosure Statement: The authors declare that they have no financial disclosures.
Division of Cardiology, University of Washington, 1959 Northeast Pacific Street Box 356422, Seattle, WA 98195, USA
* Corresponding author.
E-mail address: jmmccabe@uw.edu

Intervent Cardiol Clin 9 (2020) 41–52
https://doi.org/10.1016/j.iccl.2019.08.006

most likely to benefit from TRA access are least likely to receive TRA access.[5] Independent predictors of vascular access site complications include increased age, female sex, elevated troponin, chronic kidney disease, emergent procedures, prior PCI, diabetes, and a history of peripheral artery disease.[5] Other clinical scenarios in which TRA access may be preferred include patients on therapeutic anticoagulation, bleeding diatheses, an inability to receive transfusion or lay flat, and extremes of body mass index (BMI).[4,6,7]

In the RADIAL PUMP UP Registry, there was a significantly higher event-free survival for cardiac death, MI, target lesion revascularization, stroke, and bleeding in the population of patients who underwent single TFA access with accompanying TRA access when compared with patients who underwent bilateral TFA access.[8] Patients who undergo TRA access are also able to ambulate sooner and ultimately leads to an earlier discharge, resulting in both a reduced hospital course and shorter length of stay.[2,9,10]

Although the mortality benefit is primarily in patients who present with ACS, the increased number of access sites and larger bore equipment is likely to contribute further to procedural risk in patients who present for complex, high-risk, and indicated PCIs (CHIP). Furthermore, upper-extremity vascular access offers additional options in this complex population and is an important tool in assessing hemodynamics and implanting support devices in a subset of patients.

In this review, the authors aim to provide rationale for TRA access, describe methods to reduce access site crossover, and ultimately provide tools to help improve outcomes in patients who present for CHIP and cardiogenic shock (CS).

UPPER EXTREMITY ANATOMY

In the standard anatomic configuration, the aortic arch provides 3 major branches. From the ascending aorta those branches are the brachiocephalic trunk, the left common carotid, and the left subclavian artery.[11] The brachiocephalic trunk supplies blood to the right arm via the right subclavian artery and right head and neck via the right common carotid.[11] The left common carotid artery supplies blood to the left side of the head of the neck.[11] Lastly, the left subclavian artery distributes blood to the left arm.[11] The subclavian artery continues as the axillary artery (AA) when it emerges from under the clavicle, which in turn becomes the brachial artery before bifurcating into the ulnar

and radial arteries (RA). Typically, the RA originates within the antecubital fossa and runs down the radial side of the forearm until it reaches the wrist near the base of the thumb. From here, the main RA takes a course around the posterior aspect of the base of the thumb and first finger, where it becomes the distal or dorsal RA within the anatomic snuffbox and eventually divides into the superficial and deep palmar arches of the hand. These arches are also supplied at their opposite ends by the ulnar artery, which runs down the medial aspect of the forearm when the arm is supinated.

Several studies have evaluated the size of the RA (Table 1).[12–25] There have been significant variations in size depending on the population being studied and the method of measurement. It is thought that measurements by angiography are smaller secondary to vasoreactivity to contrast. Also, some studies administered sublingual nitroglycerin before ultrasound measurements.[15] In one of the larger studies by Yoo and colleagues,[19] the mean RA diameter was 2.60 ± 0.41 mm ($2.69 \pm .40$ in men, 2.43 ± 0.38 in women). This corresponded to 74.4% of patients (67% of men, 84.9% of women) having smaller RA diameter than the outer diameter of 7 French (Fr) sheath (2.85 mm).[19] In a second study by Saito and colleagues,[20] 40.3% of women and 71.5% of men could accommodate 7 Fr sheaths (2.85 mm). Approximately 24% of women and 44.9% of men could accommodate 8 Fr sheaths (3.22 mm).[20] When these data are interpreted in true Fr size diameter (7 Fr = 2.33 mm, 8 Fr = 2.66 mm), the number of patients that can be treated with slender and sheathless techniques increases significantly.

It is often difficult to predict which patients will have RAs compatible with larger bore access. Possible predictors of larger RA diameter include male sex, non-South Asian ancestry, and wrist circumference.[18] There has been conflicting data regarding BMI as an independent predictor of RA size. Kotowycz and colleagues[18] proposed the GRASP score, which is a scoring system to predict RA size. A score greater than or equal to 8 predicted an RA diameter greater than 2.52 mm (6 Fr sheath or 7 Fr slender/sheathless) with 100% sensitivity, 84% specificity, positive predictive value of 85%, and negative predictive value of 100%.[18]

The prevalence of RA anomalies varies significantly based on definition and population studied. They are thought to occur in as many as 13.8% of patients who present for cardiac catheterization. Anomalies of the RA, loops, or

Table 1
Radial artery size in clinical studies

Author	Country	Patients	Method	Mean diameter ± SD (mm)	Male Mean diameter ± SD (mm)	Female Mean diameter ± SD (mm)
Velasco	USA	100	Ultrasound	2.22 ± 0.35	2.42 ± 0.33	2.08 ± 0.29
Ashraf	Pakistan	251	Ultrasound	2.3 ± 0.4	-	-
Kotowycz	Canada	130	Ultrasound	2.44 ± 0.6	-	-
Yoo	South Korea	1191	Ultrasound	2.60 ± 0.41	2.69 ± .40	2.43 ± 0.38
Loh	Singapore	327	Ultrasound	2.45 ± 0.54		
Yan	China	638	Ultrasound	2.38 ± 0.56	2.47 ± 0.57	2.17 ± 0.48
Yokoyama	Japan	113	Ultrasound	2.6 ± 0.5		
Chugh	India	2344	Ultrasound	-	1.9 ± 1.12 1.7	1.7 ± 0.29
Numasawa	Japan	744	Angiography	2.69 ± 0.37	2.75 ± 0.36	2.40 ± 0.26
Gwon	South Korea	100	Angiography	3.2 ± 0.7		
Saito	Japan	250	Ultrasound	-	3.10 ± 0.60	2.80 ± 0.60
Boyer	USA	43	Angiography	2.29 ± 0.47	-	-
Baumann	USA	565	Ultrasound	3.03 ± 0.57	3.2 ± 0.56	2.7 ± 0.45

tortuosity can often be overcome with careful manipulation. However, dual RA or high branching RA are most challenging to larger sheaths and catheters (>6 Fr) as a result of a smaller caliber of the RA. These anomalies are thought to represent 7% of patients who present for catheterization and can be detected on angiogram or preprocedure ultrasound.

The dorsal or distal radial artery (DRA) access site has also recently generated interest as an access site, particularly from the patient's left hand where it provides better ergonomics. The DRA can improve both patient and physician comfort because it allows the patient's left hand to remain in a natural and neutral position throughout the entirety of the procedure.[26,27] The DRA is approximately 80% the diameter of the typical RA, measuring a mean 2.4 mm.[28] Therefore, DRA can be an additional viable access site into the arterial system.

ULTRASOUND FOR TRANSRADIAL ARTERIAL ACCESS

Many operators are comfortable obtaining arterial access by palpation for TRA. However, readily available and portable ultrasound machines are increasingly used in guiding arterial and venous access. It can be particularly useful in those patients with lower cardiac output and subsequently diminished or occasionally absent radial pulses.

As the human fingertip has a limitation of 2 to 4 mm two-point discrimination, operators may occasionally have difficulty palpating an artery with an average diameter of 2.5 to 3.0 mm.[15] A meta-analysis of randomized trials evaluating the difference in ultrasound-guided versus palpation-guided RA catheterization in adults revealed that there was a higher first-attempt success rate accompanied by a lower failure rate in the ultrasound group.[29] However, no significant difference was found in access site hematomas or time to a successful attempt.[29] Ultrasound can also be used to detect the presence of anomalies and determine sizing for equipment (sheath/guide) to prevent RA spasm.[15,24] Furthermore, there are some data to suggest the use of ultrasound can potentially decrease the risk of crossover to a different access site.[15,24]

POTENTIAL DISADVANTAGES OR CHALLENGES OF USING THE RADIAL ARTERIES

RA spasm can be challenging especially when patients have smaller RAs or when operators use larger diameter sheaths and guides. In addition, as a result of increased sheath to artery ratio, there is a possibility of causing subsequent radial artery occlusion (RAO).[20] In a small series of patients where 7- and 8-Fr guides were used for PCI, the rates of RAO were approximately 7% at 6 months of follow-up.[30,31]

RAO is often a clinically silent event and acute symptomatic RAO occurs infrequently. Nevertheless, strategies have been developed to avoid this potential outcome. These strategies include the routine use of heparin during the procedure in conjunction with antispasmolytics. In a recent study by Hahalis and colleagues,[32] there was a dose-response effect between heparin and RAO. Out of a total of 3102 patients (of whom 1836 did not receive PCI), follow-up ultrasound demonstrated a total of 102 early RAOs (incidence 5.6%). In the high-dose heparin group (100 IU/kg), the rate of RAO was significantly lower compared with the standard-dose heparin group (50 IU/kg) (27 [3.0%] vs 75 [8.1%]). The time to achieve hemostasis was similar between groups.[32]

There is also the risk for RA dissection and/or perforation. Operators should always be cognizant of wire location and never force a wire, catheter, or guide when resistance is felt. If an RA perforation does occur, an attempt to pass a 0.014" coronary wire can be made and, if successful, the diagnostic or guiding catheter can be advanced and left in place to seal the perforation while the planned procedure is continued. If hemostasis is not obtained with the catheter or guide in place, one recommendation is to inflate a manual blood pressure cuff to approximately 15 mm Hg higher than the patients' systolic blood pressure and apply a compression dressing at the site.[33] Close monitoring for signs or symptoms of compartment syndrome is required, including worsening edema, pain with passive wrist flexion, decreased sensation, or difficulty in moving fingers.[33] Evidence of compartment syndrome should prompt a vascular surgery consultation for additional assistance.

TRANSRADIAL ARTERIAL ACCESS—TIPS AND TRICKS FOR SUCCESS

There are several techniques to allow for successful advancement of guiding catheters through the RA, which are particularly helpful since crossover from the RA carries an increased risk of bleeding, increased fluoroscopic times, and ultimately inferior patient outcomes.[34] Options include, but are not limited to, the use of balloon-assisted tracking (BAT), plus dedicated devices such as telescoping or shuttle sheath, the use of sheathless guides, and the Railway system.

BAT is a method of effectively advancing a guiding catheter through a smaller diameter RA, which has increased tortuosity or friction secondary to spasm or atherosclerosis.[35] In these situations, an operator can use a 2.0 mm × 15 to 20 mm compliant rapid-

exchange angioplasty balloon over a coronary wire to the tip of their guiding catheter (Fig. 1).[35] The operator should keep the distal two-thirds of the balloon outside the guide and inflate just greater than nominal inflation pressure. The catheter and inflated balloon are then advanced as one unit where the balloon acts as a dilator for the catheter. This will allow easier advancement to the ascending aorta and eliminates the concern for the razor effect, which can result in dissection of perforation of the RA.[35,36]

Telescoping with the radial sheath in place and "homemade" sheathless guides often consist of a larger guide catheter with a smaller diameter diagnostic catheter telescoped inside of it (usually 2 Fr sizes smaller than the guide catheter and 125 cm in length—pigtail or multipurpose). This provides a more tapered end that can be advanced through the RA, without the use of a sheath, until it reaches the ascending aorta as a single unit.[37] The smaller diagnostic catheter is then removed and the guide is then advanced as usual into the coronary ostium. However, the unevenness of the transition sites between the outer edge of the guide and the outer edge of the catheter can be a culprit for resistance and vascular damage.[37,38]

As a result of telescoping and homemade sheathless guides, Asahi Intecc Co Ltd. (Aichi, Japan) designed a line of sheathless guiding catheters called the Eaucath. These guiding catheters have smooth transitions between the catheter and an inner dilator and subsequently the inner dilator and a 0.035-inch wire, thus ameliorating concerns for the razor effect.[39] The guide exterior, when kept wet, is hydrophilic, allowing a smooth entry and subsequent advancement to the aorta via the RA.[39] The Eaucath guiding catheter is available in both 6.5 and 7.5 Fr sizes with approximately 0.07" and 0.081"

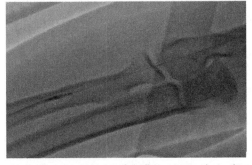

Fig. 1. Demonstration of balloon-assisted tracking with a 6-Fr EBU 3.5 guide and a 2.5 × 15 mm rapid exchange over a balloon 0.014" coronary wire.

internal diameters, respectively, and outer diameters slightly smaller than a standard 5 or 6 Fr sheath, respectively.[37,39] These guides are slightly more labor intensive if a patient has multivessel disease requiring multiple guides. And although the caliber and lubricity of the Eaucath make it an excellent option for troubleshooting RA spasm and advancing the catheter to the ascending aorta, there are concerns regarding catheter stability and support during complex PCI.[30]

An alternative to the abovementioned options is the Cordis (Santa Clara, CA) Railway system, which again eliminates the need of an access sheath. The Railway effectively acts as an introducer and stylet inside the operator's coronary catheter of choice, thereby making any catheter feasible as a sheathless option by creating a generally seamless transition between the 0.035-inch wire and catheter.

TRANSRADIAL ARTERIAL ACCESS FOR COMPLEX/HIGH-RISK PERCUTANEOUS CORONARY INTERVENTIONS AND CHRONIC TOTAL OCCLUSIONS

Many patients with complex coronary disease also have significant peripheral vascular disease, which may limit or even inhibit femoral artery access. Furthermore, if dual access sites are required for PCI, such as with chronic total occlusion (CTO) interventions, bleeding complications are intuitively increased when both femoral arteries are accessed. As operators become increasingly facile using TRA access for non-CTO PCI, many CTO operators are transitioning to single or dual TRA access to obtain the same benefits for this particular patient population. The National Database for the British Cardiovascular Interventions Society reported data on 26,807 procedures from 2006 to 2013 demonstrating that TFA had decreased from 84.5% to 57.9%.[40] Data from many case presentations and observational studies have demonstrated successful CTO recanalization using antegrade or retrograde approaches via TRA access in conjunction with reduced access site vascular complications.[41,42]

Probably the most difficult aspect of using the RA for CTOs is the desire to use 8-Fr catheters and concerns over RA size. Use of larger guides allows increased passive support for crossing complex lesions and facilitates the full range of equipment and techniques. Most contemporary observational data are from CTO PCI operators using smaller guides (<7 Fr) via TRA although advances in radial-specific sheath technology increasingly provide the opportunity to use 7-Fr guides from the radial artery or sheathless 7.5-Fr guides.[37] Typically, when one smaller and one larger guide are used for dual guided intervention (eg, a 6-Fr guide from the wrist and an 8-Fr guide from the femoral), the larger is used as the antegrade guide and the smaller is used as the retrograde guide.

There has been conflicting data regarding procedural and radiation dose using TRA access for CTO PCI.[43–45] However, as operators gain more experience and increased comfort with TRA access, their ability to perform successful CTOs through this approach has also increased.[46] Tanaka and colleagues[47] evaluated CTO PCI outcomes between TRA and TFA access and found that the use of guiding catheters smaller than 7 Fr via TRA access was a predictor of failure (odds ratio: 5.50; $P = .008$). More contemporary CTO PCI data have not shown a significant difference in success rates based on access site with the obvious caveat that such data are nonrandomized and undoubtedly confounded by selection bias.[43–45]

In a small study by Dautov and colleagues,[30] a biradial approach was used to perform CTO PCI in 110 patients via a homemade sheathless 8-Fr guide system. The patients were selected based on palpation of the RA and ostial CTOs were excluded. Their technical success rate was 93% without any major bleeding or vascular complications.[30] In addition, there was no significant increase in procedure time, contrast use, or use of radiation when compared with TFA.[30] Among the patients who had follow-up ultrasounds between 3 and 6 months, the rate of RAO was 7.1%.[30]

In the PROGRESS CTO Trial, TRA access was used in 42% of cases (either radial only or radial/femoral combination).[45] TRA access was used exclusively in 19.7% of cases. RA CTO PCI cases had lower J-CTO and PROGRESS CTO scores, smaller sheath sizes, and lower frequency of antegrade dissection reentry technique.[45] Although there were no significant differences in technical/procedural success rates or in-hospital complications, there was a statistically significant reduction in major bleeding in cases that used TRA access.[45]

In regard to left main (LM) interventions, the EXCEL trial evaluated the difference in a TFA versus TRA access.[48] EXCEL was a prospective, international, open-label, multicenter trial that randomized 1905 patients with LM disease and SYNTAX scores less than or equal to 32 to PCI with everolimus-eluting stents versus coronary artery bypass grafting.[48] Syntax score was equivalent among the TRA and TFA groups, but the TRA patients had lower rates of hypertension and chronic kidney disease as they tended to be younger.[48] Ultimately, patients undergoing TRA and TFA had similar 30-day rates of thrombolysis in myocardial infarction major or minor bleeding (2.4% vs 3.8%, respectively, $P = .30$). At 3 years, TRA and TFA patients had similar rates of the primary composite endpoint (15.7% vs 14.8%, adjusted hazard ratio 1.11, 95% confidence interval: 0.73–1.69, $P = .64$), as well as the individual rates of death, MI, stroke, ischemia-driven revascularization, and stent thrombosis.[48] In summary, TRA access was associated with similar early and late clinical outcomes when compared with TFA access for LM PCI.[48] These findings were further supported by a recent meta-analysis of nonrandomized trials comparing TRA and TFA for LM PCI by Yicong and colleagues. Their analysis found comparable MACEs between the 2 groups, but TRA access was associated with less bleeding.[49]

The use of the rotablator rotational atherectomy system (Boston Scientific, Inc, Marlborough, MA, USA) and the orbital atherectomy system (OAS) (Cardiovascular Systems, Inc., St. Paul, MN, USA) are extremely helpful when attempting to modify heavily calcified coronary lesions. The Rotoblator burr comes in several sizes. The 1.25 mm, 1.5 mm, and 1.75 mm burr will fit through most 6-Fr guiding catheters, although the 1.75 mm is much more easily delivered through a 7 Fr system. The 2.0 mm burr would require an 8-Fr guiding catheter.[50] The OAS crown is one size, 1.25 mm, and is able to be advanced into the coronary system via a 6-Fr guiding system.[51] It can also fit through a 6-Fr guide extender. Overall, both rotational and orbital atherectomy can be performed via TRA.

CARDIOGENIC SHOCK AND TRANSRADIAL ARTERIAL ACCESS

CS continues to be a leading cause of mortality in patients who present with an acute MI.[52] The ultimate goal is to restore flow in the infarct-related artery and perfusion to ischemic organs within the shortest duration of time.[53] Patients who are emergently taken to the cardiac catheterization laboratory secondary to CS are often prepped and draped for bilateral groin access if the plan is to place a percutaneous left ventricular assist device, such as Impella, extracorporeal membrane oxygenation (ECMO), or Tandem. However, many of the recent studies would advise assessing RA pulses. A meta-analysis of studies assessing patients with

cardiogenic shock found that those who were accessed via the TRA had a significantly decreased mortality rate along with lower rates of ischemia and bleeding complications when compared with TFA.[54]

The use of ultrasound is encouraged when obtaining access in CS. This can be particularly helpful as the pulse may not be palpable. TRA access remains particularly important in this population as demonstrated by Bernat and colleagues[52] who evaluated the clinical outcomes in 2663 patients who presented with STEMI, of which 197 were in CS before undergoing primary PCI. At 1 year, there was a significantly lower mortality rate for the TRA group at 44% compared with the TFA group at 64%.[52] A systematic review and meta-analysis by Pancholy and colleagues[55] further strengthen the use of TRA in patients with CS. They evaluated 8 studies involving 8131 patients, of which 5810 were included. They found TRA to be associated with a significant reduction in mortality and MACCE at 30 days.[55] Many operators will argue that obtaining TRA access may take longer in such situations as CS, but Bernat and colleagues[52] reported no difference in total ischemic time, procedural time, contrast volume use, or fluoroscopic times. To further emphasize this point, Wimmer and colleagues[56] sought to quantify the delay in reperfusion from obtaining TRA access ("transradial delay") compared with TFA access and subsequently performing a PCI in regard to patient mortality. They ultimately found that a substantial transradial delay (>80 minutes) is required to eliminate the mortality benefit observed with TRA PCI in randomized controlled trials.[56]

In the United Kingdom, many operators preferentially use TFA access for patients presenting in CS. However, a recent study of patients with high-risk CS by Mamas and colleagues[57] had similar findings as previously mentioned, including lower 30-day mortality, in-hospital major adverse cardiac and cerebrovascular events, and major bleeding.

However, one does need to be cautious when relying on observational data, particularly in the CS population. In fact, a recent analysis by Wimmer and colleagues[58] used a "falsification hypothesis" as a mechanism to explore potential residual confounding in an observational analysis of TRA versus TFA access. Conceptually, a falsification endpoint is a clinical endpoint that one would not expect to be different between the 2 cohorts studied if satisfactory statistical adjustment has been performed but is also an endpoint that could meaningfully affect outcomes. In this case, for example, non–access-related bleeding was used. If a falsification outcome is different between the 2 groups, one should necessarily be concerned about residual confounding between the populations studied despite statistical adjustment and that is just what they found in their analysis.

When hemodynamic support is required in CS, TRA access can be used to perform angiography to determine if large bore access is feasible within the axillary or iliofemoral artery. TRA access can also be used to safely obtain hemostasis if hemodynamic support is no longer needed at both the AA and TFA access sites. In several observational studies, operators have been successful at performing above-knee procedures successfully through a 6- or 7-Fr TRA system.[59,60] This can be extrapolated to operators preforming dry closure of AA or TFA access. Dry closure through the TRA access allows the operator to control hemostasis at the AA or TFA access site by balloon tamponade and can allow time for placement of a vascular closure device. If necessary, the TRA access can also be used to perform bailout stenting and provide a conduit for bypass for occlusive sheath management when a large bore sheath is left in place.[61]

CARDIOGENIC SHOCK AND AXILLARY ACCESS

The AA is increasingly used for large-bore arterial access and offers several advantages to femoral access in patients with shock requiring hemodynamic support.[62,63] First, atherosclerotic disease burden may make TFA access high risk for occlusion with indwelling large-bore catheters, cause vascular injury during implantation, or may lead to failure to obtain large-bore access and device implantation if alternative routes are not available to the operator. Second, bed rest required with an indwelling femoral catheter carries added morbidity.[64] Mobilization and vascular access options are particularly important in the CS

population, as temporary hemodynamic support devices are often used for greater than 24 hours and multiple access options may be required for additional percutaneous valvular or coronary interventions. Patients evaluated with CT angiography for transcatheter aortic valve replacement were noted to have slightly smaller caliber AA as compared with the femoral artery, with a mean size of 6.0 to 6.45 mm but less than 10% demonstrating moderate to severe calcification or stenosis in the AA as compared with 64% burden in the iliofemoral arteries.[65,66] This relative sparing of the AA from obstructive atherosclerotic disease and often adequate size for large-bore access, coupled with the ability of patients to ambulate with indwelling AA catheters, render this a particularly attractive access site in patients presenting with CS if adequate AA caliber is present.

Percutaneous AA access has been previously described and is depicted in **Fig. 2**.[63,67,68] After an operator has made the decision to use the AA for access, preprocedural imaging by ultrasound, CTA, or angiography can be extremely helpful.[69] It is recommended to use ultrasound guidance with a micropuncture kit and subsequently enter the vessel at a shallow angle with the needle.[69] Left axillary access is often best, as it avoids traversing the common carotid directly and less frequently requires managing a retroflexed angle as may be the case from the right axillary in a type I arch. A demonstration of left AA access with Impella is demonstrated in **Fig. 3**. Extrapolating from the transcatheter aortic valve replacement population, stroke may have an increased signal as compared with transaortic and transapical approaches, although this was predominantly in surgical cut down scenarios.[70,71] Although implants up to 14 Fr have become routine, larger cannula such as the one required for ECMO and the current Impella 5.0 device have not reproducibly been placed percutaneously via the AA.

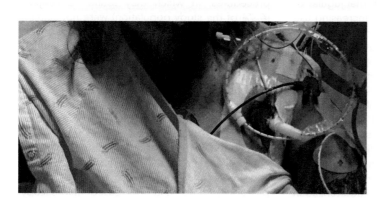

Fig. 2. Patient postprocedure with an Impella CP placed via axillary artery allowing early ambulation. (*Courtesy of* Abiomed, Danvers, MA.)

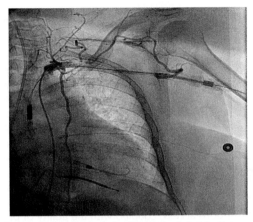

Fig. 3. Left-sided Impella CP via the left AA. Patency of the vessel is confirmed on angiography, although even if thrombus develops with prolonged use, the arm is well collateralized and ischemic symptoms are rare. (*Courtesy of* Abiomed, Danvers, MA.)

Closure of the AA arteriotomy is often cited as a concern, but cadaveric models and growing clinical experience have demonstrated that this site is in fact compressible, although hemostasis is typically facilitated via Perclose closure devices.[62,63,67] Covered stent placement is only required in rare cases for severe bleeding. Bleeding complications in this area seem rare, with no reported cases of direct hemothorax.

The decision to implant temporary hemodynamic support in CS is always a difficult balance of risks and efforts to stabilize the patient, but with growing expertise in AA access and management, this offers a distinct advantage in caring for this complex population.

ALTERNATIVE LOCATIONS FOR RIGHT HEART CATHETERIZATIONS—TIPS AND TRICKS FOR SUCCESS

Typically, most operators will perform right heart catheterizations (RHC) via the internal jugular or femoral veins. However, with the increasing use of TRA access, many operators prefer to stay in the arm if possible. Therefore, the use of the antecubital vein has grown in popularity and is more comfortable and pleasant for patients than typical access sites.

Advantages of the antecubital vein include, but are not limited to, improved patient safety, improved patient comfort, low risk of harm, no need to hold anticoagulation, earlier ambulation, and same day discharge.[72–74] In addition, patients may have their access obtained before being brought into the cardiac catheterization

laboratory, allowing busy laboratories to remain efficient.[54,74]

Ideally, the most accessible and largest antecubital vein (preferably medial or central location) should be accessed by an anterior wall stick if possible.[72] Tourniquets can be helpful in obtaining initial venous access within this vein. Successful venipuncture and advancement of sheath and RHC have been performed in veins that are greater than or equal to 6 mm in diameter (3–6 mm is borderline size) and depth should not exceed 10 mm (10–16 mm depth is borderline).[72] Once venipuncture is performed and venous blood return is observed, the 0.018-inch, 45 cm-long, soft-tipped wire (present in most radial kits) can be advanced through the needle into the proximal venous system.[72] The radial thin-walled hydrophilic 5-Fr sheaths are often useful in this location. If resistance is felt, manipulation of the wire under fluoroscopy may be advantageous as the wire may have been advanced into a small branch or may be abutting a venous valve. Transitioning to a coronary wire may also be helpful and often results in advancement to the superior vena cava via the median or cephalic veins with minimal effort.[74] If there is resistance while advancing the RHC, the operator can consider venogram for roadmap. Again, a coronary (0.014 mm) or peripheral (0.018 mm) wire can be used in addition to patient-directed instructions such as deep breaths and increased French size for more pushability (ie, 6-Fr catheter).[73–76] In cases of tortuosity or acute angulations, a 4- or 5-Fr JR 4 catheter may allow torquability to direct the wire in the correct direction and/or advance more easily. Once in the right heart, the catheter may be exchanged for a Swan-Ganz catheter over an exchange length stiff body coronary wire.

Roule and colleagues[73] evaluated their procedural outcomes during 1007 consecutive RHC procedures, in which they found 43 subjects (4.3% of the study population) were not suitable for antecubital venous access. Of the 964 patients of whom the RHC was attempted via the antecubital venous access, only 80.7% had RHC completed via the initial antecubital venous access site, making the failure rate 16.7%.[73] Of those which were unsuccessful, 8.1% had crossover to the contralateral antecubital venous access site and 6.9% crossed over to femoral vein access.[73] When using the antecubital vein, Shah and colleagues,[76] Williams and colleagues,[75] and Roule and colleagues[73] found decreased procedure time and decreased fluoroscopy.

There was also a noted decrease in complications by Gilchrist and colleagues[74] and Williams and colleagues[75] when the antecubital vein was used for RHC.

Although few, there are some disadvantages to using the antecubital vein. The patient's height is an important aspect because most RHC are only 110 cm and therefore may be difficult to reach the wedge position if the patient is extremely tall.[72] In addition, fluoroscopy use may be needed to follow the path from the antecubital fossa to the right heart.[72,77] Of note, the subclavian vein provides an additional venous access site that has been found to have a lower risk of infection and thrombosis risk,[77] albeit with an increased risk for causing pneumothorax, when compared with either the femoral, jugular, or antecubital veins.[77]

SUMMARY

As evidenced by the many observational studies, registries, and trials, TRA access is a safe and viable option for the multitude of patients and cases seen across the spectrum of coronary artery disease. Overall, TRA access results in improved outcomes, including decreased bleeding and vascular complications. TRA access also provides the patients with the ability to ambulate sooner and potentially be discharged earlier. TRA access should at least be attempted when patients present for high-risk PCI, CTO interventions, and even in the state of CS.

If the RA is difficult to palpate, use of ultrasound can always be helpful and informative regarding the course of the RA and highlight areas of concern. In addition, there are many ways to prevent crossover in smaller diameter RA or tortuous RA such as telescoping, BAT, or sheathless guides.

Axillary arterial access offers advantages for large bore access when required for hemodynamic support in CS or other invasive procedures. Patient mobility with an indwelling device and relative sparing of the axillary arteries from atherosclerotic and calcific disease as compared with the iliac and femoral arteries makes this a great choice for indwelling device therapy.

Finally, if right heart pressures are desired during the time of a cardiac catheterization, the antecubital vein is a viable option into the venous system. It allows the operator to remain in one access site location when using the RA and again has decreased complications with improved patient comfort.

REFERENCES

1. Ferrante G, Rao SV, Jüni P, et al. Radial versus femoral access for coronary interventions across the entire spectrum of patients with coronary artery disease. JACC Cardiovasc Interv 2016;9(14):1419–34.
2. Jolly SS, Yusuf S, Cairns J, et al. Radial versus femoral access for coronary angiography and intervention in patients with acute coronary syndromes (RIVAL): a randomised, parallel group, multicentre trial. Lancet 2011;377(9775):1409–20.
3. Neumann F-J, Sousa-Uva M, Ahlsson A, et al. 2018 ESC/EACTS Guidelines on myocardial revascularization. Eur Heart J 2019;40(2):87–165.
4. Mason PJ, Shah B, Tamis-Holland JE, et al. An update on radial artery access and best practices for transradial coronary angiography and intervention in acute coronary syndrome: a scientific statement from the American Heart Association. Circ Cardiovasc Interv 2018;11(9). https://doi.org/10.1161/HCV.0000000000000035.
5. Wimmer NJ, Resnic FS, Mauri L, et al. Risk-treatment paradox in the selection of transradial access for percutaneous coronary intervention. J Am Heart Assoc 2013;2(3). https://doi.org/10.1161/JAHA.113.000174.
6. Brueck M, Bandorski D, Kramer W, et al. A randomized comparison of transradial versus transfemoral approach for coronary angiography and angioplasty. JACC Cardiovasc Interv 2009;2(11):1047–54.
7. Baker NC, O'Connell EW, Htun WW, et al. Safety of coronary angiography and percutaneous coronary intervention via the radial versus femoral route in patients on uninterrupted oral anticoagulation with warfarin. Am Heart J 2014;168(4):537–44.
8. Romagnoli E, De Vita M, Burzotta F, et al. Radial versus femoral approach comparison in percutaneous coronary intervention with intraaortic balloon pump support: the RADIAL PUMP UP Registry Background The role of intraaortic balloon pump (IABP) during percutaneous coronary intervention (PCI) in high-risk. Am Heart J 2013;166:1019–26.
9. Pristipino C, Trani C, Nazzaro MS, et al. Major improvement of percutaneous cardiovascular procedure outcomes with radial artery catheterisation: results from the PREVAIL study in the Lazio region, the second most Interventional cardiology. Heart 2009;95:476–82.
10. Mann T, Cubeddu G, Bowen J, et al, CLINICAL STUDIES INTERVENTIONAL CARDIOLOGY. Stenting in acute coronary syndromes: a comparison of radial versus femoral access sites. J Am Coll Cardiol 1998. https://doi.org/10.1016/S0735-1097(98)00288-5.
11. Kelley JD, Ashurst JV. Anatomy, thorax, aortic arch 2019. Available at: https://www.ncbi.nlm.nih.gov/books/NBK499911/. Accessed May 19, 2019.

12. Velasco A, Ono C, Nugent K, et al. Ultrasonic evaluation of the radial artery diameter in a local population from Texas. J Invasive Cardiol 2012;24(7): 339–41. Available at: http://www.ncbi.nlm.nih.gov/pubmed/22781473. Accessed April 28, 2019.

13. Ashraf T, Panhwar Z, Habib S, et al. Size of radial and ulnar artery in local population. J Pak Med Assoc 2010;60(10):817–9. Available at: http://www.ncbi.nlm.nih.gov/pubmed/21381609. Accessed April 28, 2019.

14. Gwon HC, Doh JH, Choi JH, et al. A 5Fr catheter approach reduces patient discomfort during transradial coronary intervention compared with a 6Fr approach: a prospective randomized study. J Interv Cardiol 2006;19(2):141–7.

15. Baumann F, Roberts JS. Real time intraprocedural ultrasound measurements of the radial and ulnar arteries in 565 consecutive patients undergoing cardiac catheterization and/or percutaneous coronary intervention via the wrist: understanding anatomy and anomalies may improve acce. J Interv Cardiol 2015;28(6):574–82.

16. Dharma S, Kedev S, Patel T, et al. Radial artery diameter does not correlate with body mass index: a duplex ultrasound analysis of 1706 patients undergoing trans-radial catheterization at three experienced radial centers. Int J Cardiol 2016. https://doi.org/10.1016/j.ijcard.2016.11.145.

17. Nagai S, Abe S, Sato T, et al. Ultrasonic assessment of vascular complications in coronary angiography and angioplasty after transradial approach. Am J Cardiol 1999;83(2):180–6. Available at: http://www.ncbi.nlm.nih.gov/pubmed/10073818. Accessed April 28, 2019.

18. Kotowycz MA, Johnston KW, Ivanov J, et al. Predictors of radial artery size in patients undergoing cardiac catheterization: insights from the good radial artery size prediction (GRASP) study. Can J Cardiol 2014;30:211–6.

19. Yoo BS, Yoon J, Ko JY, et al. Anatomical consideration of the radial artery for transradial coronary procedures: arterial diameter, branching anomaly and vessel tortuosity. Int J Cardiol 2004. https://doi.org/10.1016/j.ijcard.2004.03.061.

20. Saito S, Ikei H, Hosokawa G, et al. Influence of the ratio between radial artery inner diameter and sheath outer diameter on radial artery flow after transradial coronary intervention. Catheter Cardiovasc Interv 1999;46(2):173–8.

21. Yan Z, Zhou Y, Zhao Y, et al. Anatomical study of forearm arteries with ultrasound for percutaneous coronary procedures. Circ J 2010;74(4):686–92. Available at: http://www.ncbi.nlm.nih.gov/pubmed/20197630. Accessed April 28, 2019.

22. Loh YJ, Nakao M, Tan WD, et al. Factors influencing radial artery size. Asian Cardiovasc Thorac Ann 2007;15(4):324–6.

23. Yokoyama N, Takeshita S, Ochiai M, et al. Anatomic variations of the radial artery in patients undergoing transradial coronary intervention. Catheter Cardiovasc Interv 2000;49(4):357–62.

24. Kumar Chugh S, Chugh S, Chugh Y, et al. Feasibility and utility of pre-procedure ultrasound imaging of the arm to facilitate transradial coronary diagnostic and interventional procedures (PRIMA-FACIE-TRI). Catheter Cardiovasc Interv 2013;82(1): 64–73.

25. Boyer N, Beyer A, Gupta V, et al. The effects of intra-arterial vasodilators on radial artery size and spasm: implications for contemporary use of trans-radial access for coronary angiography and percutaneous coronary intervention. Cardiovasc Revasc Med 2013;14:321–4.

26. Davies RE, Gilchrist IC. Back hand approach to radial access: the snuff box approach. Cardiovasc Revasc Med 2018;19(3 Pt B):324–6.

27. Davies RE, Gilchrist IC. Dorsal (distal) transradial access for coronary angiography and intervention. Interv Cardiol Clin 2019. https://doi.org/10.1016/j.iccl.2018.11.002.

28. Hull JE, Kinsey EN, Bishop WL. Mapping of the snuffbox and cubital vessels for percutaneous arterial venous fistula (pAVF) in dialysis patients. J Vasc Access 2013;14(3):245–51.

29. Pacha HM, Alahdab F, Al-Khadra Y, et al. Ultrasound-guided versus palpation-guided radial artery catheterization in adult population: a systematic review and meta-analysis of randomized controlled trials. Am Heart J 2018. https://doi.org/10.1016/j.ahj.2018.06.007.

30. Dautov R, Ribeiro HB, Altisent A-J, et al. Effectiveness and safety of the transradial 8Fr sheathless approach for revascularization of chronic total occlusions. Am J Cardiol 2016. https://doi.org/10.1016/j.amjcard.2016.06.052.

31. Tumscitz C, Pirani L, Tebaldi M, et al. Seven french radial artery access for PCI: a prospective single-center experience. Int J Cardiol 2014;176(3): 1074–5.

32. Hahalis GN, Leopoulou M, Tsigkas G, et al. Multicenter randomized evaluation of high versus standard heparin dose on incident radial arterial occlusion after transradial coronary angiography. JACC Cardiovasc Interv 2018;11(22):2241–50.

33. Tizon MH, Barbeau GR. Incidence of compartment syndrome of the arm in a large series of transradial approach for coronary procedures. J Interv Cardiol 2008;21(5):380–4.

34. Le J, Bangalore S, Guo Y, et al. Predictors of access site crossover in patients who underwent transradial coronary angiography. Am J Cardiol 2015. https://doi.org/10.1016/j.amjcard.2015.04.051.

35. Patel T, Shah S, Pancholy S. Balloon-assisted tracking of a guide catheter through difficult radial

anatomy: a technical report. Catheter Cardiovasc Interv 2013;81(5):E215–8.

36. Patel T, Shah S, Pancholy S, et al. Balloon-assisted tracking: a must-know technique to overcome difficult anatomy during transradial approach. Catheter Cardiovasc Interv 2014; 83(2):211–20.

37. Gilchrist IC, Awuor SO, Davies RE, et al. Controversies in complex percutaneous coronary intervention: radial versus femoral. Expert Rev Cardiovasc Ther 2017;15(9):695–704.

38. Abdelaal E, Rimac G, Plourde G, et al. 4Fr in 5Fr sheathless technique with standard catheters for transradial coronary interventions: technical challenges and persisting issues. Catheter Cardiovasc Interv 2015;85(5):809–15.

39. Gilchrist IC. Sheathless guide catheters during transradial PCI Bigger catheters in smaller spaces. Card Interv Today 2016. Available at: https://citoday.com/2016/10/sheathless-guide-catheters-during-transradial-pci?center=134. Accessed April 28, 2019.

40. Kinnaird T, Anderson R, Ossei-Gerning N, et al. Vascular access site and outcomes among 26,807 chronic total coronary occlusion angioplasty cases from the british cardiovascular interventions society national database. JACC Cardiovasc Interv 2017; 10(7):635–44.

41. Rathore S, Hakeem A, Pauriah M, et al. A comparison of the transradial and the transfemoral approach in chronic total occlusion percutaneous coronary intervention. Catheter Cardiovasc Interv 2009;73(7):883–7.

42. Rinfret S, Joyal D, Nguyen CM, et al. Retrograde recanalization of chronic total occlusions from the transradial approach; early canadian experience. Catheter Cardiovasc Interv 2011;78(3). https://doi.org/10.1002/ccd.23140.

43. Alaswad K, Menon RV, Christopoulos G, et al. Transradial approach for coronary chronic total occlusion interventions: insights from a contemporary multicenter registry. Catheter Cardiovasc Interv 2015;85(7):1123–9.

44. Bakker EJ, Maeremans J, Zivelonghi C, et al. Fully transradial versus transfemoral approach for percutaneous intervention of coronary chronic total occlusions applying the hybrid algorithm. Circ Cardiovasc Interv 2017;10(9). https://doi.org/10.1161/CIRCINTERVENTIONS.117.005255.

45. Tajti P, Alaswad K, Karmpaliotis D, et al. Procedural outcomes of percutaneous coronary interventions for chronic total occlusions via the radial approach: insights from an international chronic total occlusion registry. JACC Cardiovasc Interv 2019;12(4): 346–58.

46. Burzotta F, De Vita M, Lefevre T, et al. Radial approach for percutaneous coronary interventions on chronic total occlusions: Technical issues and data review. Catheter Cardiovasc Interv 2014; 83(1):47–57.

47. Tanaka Y, Moriyama N, Ochiai T, et al. Transradial coronary interventions for complex chronic total occlusions. JACC Cardiovasc Interv 2017;10(3): 235–43.

48. Chen S, Redfors B, Liu Y, et al. Radial versus femoral artery access in patients undergoing PCI for left main coronary artery disease: analysis from the EXCEL trial. EuroIntervention 2018;14(10): 1104–11.

49. Ye Y, Zeng Y. Comparison between radial and femoral access for percutaneous coronary intervention in left main coronary artery disease. Coron Artery Dis 2019;30(2):79–86.

50. Tomey MI, Kini AS, Sharma SK. Current status of rotational atherectomy. JACC Cardiovasc Interv 2014;7(4):345–53.

51. Ruisi M, Zachariah J, Ratcliffe J. Safety and feasibility of the coronary orbital atherectomy system via the transradial approach | journal of invasive cardiology. 2015. Available at: https://www.invasivecardiology.com/articles/safety-and-feasibility-coronary-orbital-atherectomy-system-transradial-approach. Accessed April 28, 2019.

52. Bernat I, Abdelaal E, Plourde G, et al. Early and late outcomes after primary percutaneous coronary intervention by radial or femoral approach in patients presenting in acute ST-elevation myocardial infarction and cardiogenic shock. Background Although radial approach is increasingly used in per. Am Heart J 2013. https://doi.org/10.1016/j.ahj.2013.01.012.

53. Hochman JS, Sleeper LA, Webb JG, et al. Early revascularization in acute myocardial infarction complicated by cardiogenic shock. N Engl J Med 1999;341(9):625–34.

54. Roule V, Lemaitre A, Sabatier R, et al. Transradial versus transfemoral approach for percutaneous coronary intervention in cardiogenic shock: a radial-first centre experience and meta-analysis of published studies. Arch Cardiovasc Dis 2015; 108(11):563–75.

55. Pancholy SB, Palamaner G, Shantha S, et al. Impact of access site choice on outcomes of patients with cardiogenic shock undergoing percutaneous coronary intervention: a systematic review and meta-analysis. Am Heart J 2015. https://doi.org/10.1016/j.ahj.2015.05.001.

56. Wimmer NJ, Cohen DJ, Wasfy JH, et al. Delay in reperfusion with transradial percutaneous coronary intervention for ST-elevation myocardial infarction: might some delays be acceptable? Am Heart J 2014;168(1):103–9.

57. Mamas MA, Anderson SG, Ratib K, et al. Arterial access site utilization in cardiogenic shock in the United Kingdom: Is radial access feasible?

Background Cardiogenic shock (CS) remains the leading cause of mortality in patients hospitalized with acute. Am Heart J 2014;167:900–8.e1.

58. Wimmer NJ, Resnic FS, Mauri L, et al. Comparison of transradial versus transfemoral percutaneous coronary intervention in routine practice: evidence for the importance of "falsification hypotheses" in observational studies of comparative effectiveness. J Am Coll Cardiol 2013;62(22):2147–8.

59. Cortese B, Trani C, Lorenzoni R, et al. Safety and feasibility of iliac endovascular interventions with a radial approach. Results from a multicenter study coordinated by the Italian Radial Force. Int J Cardiol 2014;175(2):280–4.

60. Sanghvi K, Kurian D, Coppola J. Transradial intervention of iliac and superficial femoral artery disease is feasible. J Interv Cardiol 2008;21(5):385–7.

61. Kaki A, Alraies MC, Schreiber T. The challenge of large bore occlusive sheath management: strategies for success. Cardiology Today's intervention. 2018. Available at: https://www.healio.com/cardiac-vascular-intervention/peripheral/news/print/cardiology-today-intervention/%7Be1cddc7c-49cf-42a2-a4b1-5709b79 72252%7D/the-challenge-of-large-bore-occlusive-sheath-management-strategies-for-success. Accessed May 3, 2019.

62. Kaki A, Blank N, Alraies MC, et al. Axillary artery access for mechanical circulatory support devices in patients with prohibitive peripheral arterial disease presenting with cardiogenic shock. Am J Cardiol 2019;123(10):1715–21.

63. Mathur M, Hira RS, Smith BM, et al. Fully percutaneous technique for transaxillary implantation of the impella CP. JACC Cardiovasc Interv 2016; 9(11):1196–8.

64. Adler J, Malone D. Early mobilization in the intensive care unit: a systematic review. Cardiopulm Phys Ther J 2012;23(1):5. Available at: https://www.ncbi.nlm.nih.gov/pmc/articles/PMC3286494/. Accessed June 16, 2019.

65. Tayal R, Iftikhar H, LeSar B, et al. CT angiography analysis of axillary artery diameter versus common femoral artery diameter: implications for axillary approach for transcatheter aortic valve replacement in patients with hostile aortoiliac segment and advanced lung disease. Int J Vasc Med 2016; 2016:1–5.

66. Arnett DM, Lee JC, Harms MA, et al. Caliber and fitness of the axillary artery as a conduit for large-bore cardiovascular procedures. Catheter Cardiovasc Interv 2018;91(1):150–6.

67. Mathur M, Krishnan SK, Levin D, et al. A step-by-step guide to fully percutaneous transaxillary

transcatheter aortic valve replacement. Struct Hear 2017;1(5–6):209–15.

68. Schäfer U, Ho Y, Frerker C, et al. Direct percutaneous access technique for transaxillary transcatheter aortic valve implantation: "The Hamburg Sankt Georg approach." JACC Cardiovasc Interv 2012;5(5):477–86.

69. Cheney AE, McCabe JM. Alternative percutaneous access for large bore devices. Circ Cardiovasc Interv 2019;12(6). https://doi.org/10.1161/CIRCINTERVENTIONS.118.007707.

70. Dahle TG, Kaneko T, McCabe JM. Outcomes following subclavian and axillary artery access for transcatheter aortic valve replacement: Society of the Thoracic Surgeons/American College of Cardiology TVT Registry Report. JACC Cardiovasc Interv 2019;12(7):662–9.

71. McCabe J, Khaki A, Nicholson W, et al. TCT-99 safety and efficacy of percutaneous axillary artery access for mechanical circulatory support with the Impella© devices: an initial evaluation from the axillary access Registry to monitor safety (ARMS) MultiCenter Registry. J Am Coll Cardiol 2017;70(18):B43.

72. Waheed O, Sharma A, Singh M, et al. Antecubital fossa venous access for right heart catheterization. J Invasive Cardiol 2017;29(5):169–74. Available at: https://www.invasivecardiology.com/sites/invasive-cardiology.com/files/169-174 Waheed 2017 JIC May wm_0.pdf. Accessed April 13, 2019.

73. Roule V, Ailem S, Legallois D, et al. Antecubital vs femoral venous access for right heart catheterization: benefits of a flashback. Can J Cardiol 2015. https://doi.org/10.1016/j.cjca.2015.04.026.

74. Gilchrist IC, Moyer CD, Gascho JA. Transradial right and left heart catheterizations: a comparison to traditional femoral approach. Catheter Cardiovasc Interv 2006;67(4):585–8.

75. Williams P, Palmer S, Judkins C, et al. Right and left heart catheterization via an antecubital fossa vein and the radial artery – a prospective study. J Invasive Cardiol 2014;26(12):669–73. Available at: https://www.invasivecardiology.com/sites/invasive-cardiology.com/files/wm 669-673 Williams JIC Dec 2014.pdf. Accessed April 21, 2019.

76. Shah S, Boyd G, Pyne CT, et al. Right heart catheterization using antecubital venous access: feasibility, safety and adoption rate in a tertiary center. Catheter Cardiovasc Interv 2014;84(1):70–4.

77. Parienti JJ, Mongardon N, Mégarbane B, et al. Intravascular complications of central venous catheterization by insertion Site. N Engl J Med 2015; 373(13):1220–9.

Radial Access for Peripheral Interventions

Alexander C. Fanaroff, MD, MHS[a],*, Sunil V. Rao, MD[b], Rajesh V. Swaminathan, MD[b]

KEYWORDS

- Peripheral vascular intervention • Radial artery • Peripheral arterial disease

---

KEY POINTS

- Access via the radial artery is increasing for percutaneous coronary intervention and angiography because of the lower risk of vascular access and bleeding complications compared with transfemoral access.
- Peripheral vascular intervention (PVI) has traditionally been performed via transfemoral artery access because of a lack of equipment to support these procedures via the transradial approach.
- With newly developed catheters to support PVI via transradial access, the potential benefits and challenges of this approach should be reevaluated.
- Transradial access for PVI may reduce vascular access complications compared with transfemoral access, but its impact on risk of stroke, acute kidney injury, and radiation exposure during PVI needs further study.

Peripheral artery disease (PAD), defined as partial or complete obstruction of at least 1 peripheral artery, affects more than 200 million people worldwide, and is associated with substantial morbidity and health care costs.[1–3] PAD has become more prevalent, especially in the developing world, with women and younger patients increasingly affected.[4] Despite this increasing prevalence in younger patients, PAD is most common in older patients, affecting 40% of women and 30% of men more than 80 years old.[5]

Although patients may develop vascular disease in any peripheral vascular bed (cerebrovascular, mesenteric, upper extremity, lower extremity), the term PAD is usually used to describe occlusive disease in the lower extremities caused by atherosclerosis. Patients with lower extremity PAD may be asymptomatic, have intermittent claudication of varying severity, or have critical limb ischemia (CLI). Intermittent claudication is present in roughly 30% of patients with PAD, and may cause significant functional limitation.[6] Over 5-year follow-up, 5% to 10% of patients with PAD progress to CLI. CLI is characterized by rest pain, tissue loss, or gangrene, and is a highly morbid condition. Up to half of all patients with CLI undergo major amputation within 4 years of diagnosis, and 40% die within 2 years.[7,8]

Revascularization, either surgical or endovascular, improves quality of life in patients with intermittent claudication and may reduce the risk of amputation and major adverse limb events in patients with CLI.[9–12] Overall, 69% of lower extremity revascularization procedures performed in the United States are endovascular, including 78% of procedures performed for claudication and 65% of procedures performed for CLI.[13] In 97% of cases, peripheral vascular intervention (PVI) is performed via transfemoral access (TFA).[14] Access site complications, including hematoma, pseudoaneurysm formation, and

---

Disclosures: Dr A.C. Fanaroff, research support from Boston Scientific; Dr R.V. Swaminathan, research support from ACIST Medical and Cardiovascular Systems and consulting for Medtronic; Dr S.V. Rao reports no relevant disclosures.
[a] Division of Cardiology, University of Pennsylvania, Philadelphia, PA, USA; [b] Division of Cardiology, Duke Clinical Research Institute, Duke University, 200 Morris Street, Durham, NC 27701, USA
* Corresponding author. Perelman Center for Advanced Medicine, 11-103, 3400 Civic Center Boulevard, Philadelphia, PA 19104.
E-mail address: alexander.fanaroff@pennmedicine.upenn.edu

retroperitoneal hematoma, are the most common complications associated with TFA. These complications cause substantial morbidity, including hospitalization and surgical repair in some cases, and are associated with higher health care costs and an increased risk of short-term and long-term mortality.[15,16] Transradial artery access (TRA), a technique associated with a lower risk of access site complications than TFA among patients undergoing percutaneous coronary intervention (PCI),[17] has not been commonly used for PVI because of an absence of devices designed for this application. However, the safety of TRA compared with TFA, combined with an emerging collection of devices that make radial-to-peripheral procedures feasible, sets the stage for the emergence of TRA as a viable alternative to TFA for lower extremity PVI. However, several questions remain to be answered before TRA supplants TFA in PVI.

THE CASE FOR TRANSRADIAL ACCESS IN PERIPHERAL VASCULAR INTERVENTION

Among patients undergoing PCI via TFA, ~1% to 6% develop access site complications, depending on patient population and definition of access site complication.[18–20] Patients with access site complications have health care costs $6377 higher than those who do not, spend 2.8 additional days in the hospital, and are ~3-fold more likely to die over both short-term and long-term follow-up.[15,21]

PAD is one of the strongest predictors of access site complications requiring surgical intervention among patients undergoing TFA for coronary angiography or PCI; patients with PAD have a risk of access site complications requiring surgical intervention 2.5-fold higher than those without PAD, and 1.6% of patients with PAD undergoing coronary angiography via TFA develop a vascular access complication requiring surgery.[19] Moreover, some bleeding avoidance strategies may not be useful in patients with PAD. Ultrasonography-guided TFA, a technique shown to reduce vascular access complications in a randomized trial of patients undergoing coronary angiography,[22] was not specifically evaluated in patients with PAD, and its efficacy in patients undergoing PVI is uncertain.[23–25] Patients with fluoroscopically visible calcium of the common femoral artery or significant femoral artery stenosis were excluded from most trials of arterial closure devices,[26] and the effectiveness of these devices is uncertain in patients with PAD.[27] By contrast, patients with PAD were included in randomized controlled trials of TRA versus TFA in

patients undergoing coronary angiography and/or PCI. In a meta-analysis of 31 trials, TRA reduced the risk of access site complications by 64% (odds ratio, 0.36; 95% confidence interval, 0.22–0.59) among all patients; 2.7% of patients randomized to TRA had access site complications compared with 5.0% of patients randomized to TFA.[17] In MATRIX (Minimizing Adverse Haemorrhagic Events by Transradial Access Site and Systemic Implementation of Angiox), the largest trial comparing TRA and TFA in patients undergoing PCI, 713 of 8404 (8.5%) patients had PAD, and the effect of TRA on access site complications was not significantly different in patients with and without PAD.[28]

Given the higher incidence of access site complications in patients with PAD compared with those without PAD undergoing TFA for coronary angiography, it is unsurprising that PVI for lower extremity PAD is frequently complicated by vascular access complications. In an analysis of the Vascular Quality Initiative registry, 3.5% of PVI procedures (n = 936 of 27,048) were complicated by an access site complication[14]; other series have found a rate of access site complications as high as 11%.[29] Most of these access site complications are minor, but 10% require transfusion, 5% require thrombin injection, and 10% require surgical intervention (Fig. 1).[14] In the National Cardiovascular Data Registry's Peripheral Vascular Intervention Registry, compared with patients without access site complications, patients with access site complications have longer hospital stays (1.6 vs 1.2 days), are less likely to be discharged home (62.1 vs 89.1%), and have higher 30-day mortality (6.1 vs 1.4%).[14] If TRA reduces access site complications in patients undergoing PVI as it does in patients undergoing coronary angiography or PCI, then this reduction may translate into improved patient outcomes and health care costs.

TRA for PVI has several other potential benefits. Compared with TFA, TRA reduces the incidence of acute kidney injury (AKI) in patients undergoing PCI.[30] In an analysis of the National Cardiovascular Data Registry's PVI Registry, 7.4% of patients (737 of 10,006) developed AKI; in-hospital mortality was 7.0% in patients with AKI and 0.7% in those without.[31] If TRA reduces AKI in patients undergoing PVI as it does in patients undergoing PCI, this approach may also contribute to improved patient outcomes. TRA also improves patient satisfaction among patients undergoing PCI,[28] and facilitates same-day discharge by removing the need for prolonged best rest following the procedure. In addition to improving patient satisfaction,

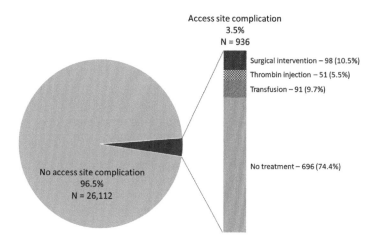

Access site complication
3.5%
N = 936

No access site complication
96.5%
N = 26,112

Surgical intervention – 98 (10.5%)
Thrombin injection – 51 (5.5%)
Transfusion – 91 (9.7%)

No treatment – 696 (74.4%)

Fig. 1. Access site complications following PVI. Of 27,048 PVIs performed from 2007 to 2013 at more than 130 sites, 936 (3.5%) had a vascular access complication. Most of these vascular access complications did not require further treatment, but 10% required surgical intervention. (*Data from* Ortiz D, Jahangir A, Singh M, et al. Access Site Complications After Peripheral Vascular Interventions. *Circ Cardiovasc Interv.* 2014;7(6):821-828.)

same-day discharge is associated with substantial cost savings.[32] Most patients undergoing PVI are already discharged on the same day as their procedure,[33] but TRA could nevertheless shorten recovery time and incrementally increase same-day discharge rates.

Another potential benefit of TRA is the potential to perform PVI on lesions in both legs through 1 access point. Via standard retrograde TFA, operators are limited to intervening on the ipsilateral iliac artery or the contralateral lower extremity. PVI of a lesion in the ipsilateral lower extremity requires a second access point in the contralateral femoral artery. Frequently, operators perform bilateral interventions in 2 separate procedures, inconveniencing the patients and exposing them to the risk of a second vascular access.

From the operator standpoint, lower extremity PVI may result in substantial radiation exposure or ergonomic challenges, especially when intervening on the right lower extremity via left femoral artery access. With a standard fluoroscopic setup and the operator positioned on the patient's right side, the operator must reach under the image intensifier to manipulate devices. Right radial access enables the operator to stand back from the image intensifier and still manipulate devices, reducing radiation exposure and the risk of orthopedic injuries. Via left radial access, adduction of the patient's arm could potentially enable a similar setup.

THE EVIDENCE BASE OF TRANSRADIAL ACCESS FOR PERIPHERAL VASCULAR INTERVENTION

To date, 19 studies including 638 patients have reported outcomes for patients undergoing lower extremity PVI via TRA; these studies have been summarized in a systematic review and meta-analysis.[34] All studies were either cohort studies, case-control studies, or case reports, and most had a small sample size (n = 1–156). Most lesions (n = 322 of 403 with lesion location reported; 79.9%) were located in the iliac arteries (**Fig. 2**A). Procedural success ranged from 81% to 100% in individual studies (mean, 90.9%), with conversion to TFA in 9.9% of cases overall (**Fig. 2**B).

The evidence for renal, visceral, and subclavian artery PVI is even scanter. Four observational studies of 87 total renal artery lesions have been published, of which procedural success was achieved in 81 (93%) without any major access site complications.[35–38] Two case series have described subclavian artery PVI via TRA in 68 patients; procedure success was achieved in 96% with crossover to femoral access in 2 patients (3.7%).[39,40] No large case series or observational studies of celiac or mesenteric artery interventions via TRA have been reported. A single-center report of 1531 noncoronary interventions performed via TRA over 3 years included 172 renal or visceral interventions and 43 PVIs.[41] Overall, technical success was achieved in 98.2% of cases, with 1.8% requiring crossover to TFA; 25 patients (1.6%) had access site complications.

Given the design of the studies (especially related to how patients were selected for TRA) and the possibility of publication bias, it is likely that the reported outcomes of lower extremity PVI via TRA in the literature are optimistic estimates of outcomes were TRA more widely implemented for PVI in clinical practice. In 1 small retrospective cohort study comparing TRA with TFA (n = 88 procedures), procedures

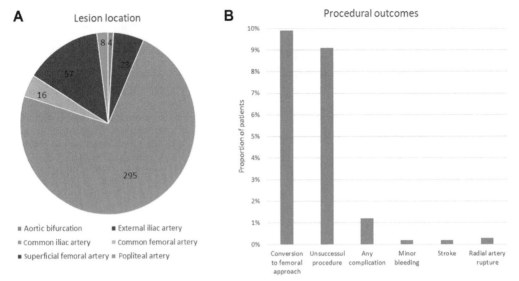

Fig. 2. Reported experience with lower extremity PVI via transradial access. A systematic review and meta-analysis identified 19 studies reporting outcomes of lower extremity PVI procedures performed via radial access. Of 19 studies, 4 were prospective cohort studies, 4 were retrospective cohort studies, 2 were case-control studies, 3 were case series, and 6 were case reports. Sample size ranged from 1 to 156. (A) Of 403 procedures with an anatomic lesion location identified, the lesion was in the iliac arteries in 322 (79.9%). (B) Across the 19 studies, conversion to a femoral approach occurred in 9.9% of procedures and 9.1% of procedures were unsuccessful. Twelve patients had any complication, including 1 each with stroke and minor bleeding, and 2 with radial artery rupture. (*Data from* Meertens MM, Ng E, Loh SEK, et al. Transradial Approach for Aortoiliac and Femoropopliteal Interventions: A Systematic Review and Meta-analysis. *J Endovasc Ther.* 2018;25(5):599-607.)

done via TRA had lower technical success, a higher rate of access site complications, and longer fluoroscopy time than procedures done via TFA.[42] In a small randomized controlled trial of TRA versus TFA for extracranial carotid artery interventions (n = 260 patients), procedure success was 100% in both arms, but 10 patients (7.7%) crossed over to TFA in the TRA group. There was no difference in the rate of major vascular access complications (1 patient in each group) and radiation dose was higher in the TRA group.[43]

BARRIERS TO AND CURRENT CHALLENGES OF TRANSRADIAL ACCESS FOR PERIPHERAL VASCULAR INTERVENTION

TRA for PVI has several challenges that may lead to conversion to TFA or unsuccessful procedures. The first challenge is related to the vascular anatomy of the upper extremity. In RIVAL (Radial vs Femoral Access for Coronary Angiography and Intervention in Patients with Acute Coronary Syndromes), a clinical trial that randomized 7021 patients undergoing PCI to TRA or TFA, 7.0% of patients assigned to TRA crossed over to TFA after a failed attempted at TRA.[44] The most common cause of crossover was radial artery spasm

(5.0%), followed by subclavian tortuosity (1.9%), and radial artery loop (1.3%). Radial artery spasm is associated with larger sheath sizes and smaller radial artery diameters.[45] Radial artery diameters range from 2 to 4 mm on radiographic, ultrasonography, and anatomic studies, with averages of 2.6 mm in men and 2.4 mm in women, smaller than the outer diameter of a 6-French (Fr) sheath (2.6–2.9 mm). The radial artery can expand beyond its resting diameter, and most patients can accommodate a 6-Fr sheath, but fewer patients may be able to tolerate larger sheaths.[46] Radial artery spasm is more than 3-fold more common in patients with PAD than in patients without,[47] likely related to endothelial dysfunction and smaller vessel lumens in patients with a high burden of systemic atherosclerosis.[45] Prolonged exposure to large-bore sheaths has been reported to cause spasm severe enough to entrap catheters in the radial artery, potentially causing severe injury to the radial artery or requiring deep sedation or axillary nerve block to safely extract devices.[46] Subclavian artery tortuosity is also more difficult to navigate in patients with calcified and atherosclerotic peripheral vasculature, although this may be less of an issue when accessing the descending thoracic aorta for PVI compared with the ascending aorta for PCI, and several strategies have been devised to overcome tortuosity.[48]

The second challenge is distance from the radial artery to the lower extremity vasculature. In a patient shorter than 178 cm (70 inches), it is roughly 110 cm from the left radial artery to the iliac bifurcation and 125 cm to the common femoral artery; distances are ~10 cm longer from the right radial artery (Fig. 3). By contrast, distance to the lesion is less of a challenge for renal, mesenteric, subclavian, or carotid interventions, which can be performed with standard-length devices because nearly all lesions are 100 cm or less from the radial artery cannulation site. Longer distances from access to lesion may complicate PVI by limiting the ability to push to cross tight lesions or if devices with long enough working length are not available. New radial-to-peripheral devices with longer working lengths are becoming available (Box 1 for a description of technical aspects of lower extremity PVI via TRA). A dedicated line of radial-to-peripheral devices, including 120-cm and 150-cm sheaths; 350-cm, 400-cm, and 450-cm 0.89-mm (0.035″) guidewires; 150-cm support microcatheters; and rapid exchange balloons with 200-cm shafts have been developed to support TRA for interventions in the iliac and superficial femoral vessels (Terumo Medical, Tokyo, Japan) (Table 1). A selection of self-expanding stents with longer shaft lengths will be available soon. Long 0.457-mm (0.018″) and 0.356-mm (0.014″) guidewires are also available from several manufacturers. An orbital atherectomy system with shaft length sufficient to treat lesions in the superficial femoral arteries via radial access has also been developed (Cardiovascular Systems, Inc., St Paul, MN).

However, the delivery of sheaths via TRA that are long and stiff enough to provide adequate support for complex superficial femoral artery PVI may be complicated in patients with PAD by radial artery spasm or stenosis in the radial, brachial, axillary, or subclavian arteries. Furthermore, device selection remains limited: there are no drug-coated balloons or smaller-diameter drug-eluting stents with shafts long enough for use via TRA. Stents will only be available in diameters of 6 to 8 mm, which is likely to be adequate in most, but not all, patients. In the event of a severe perforation, covered stents with appropriate shaft lengths and sheath size (5 or 6 Fr) compatibility for use in the iliac and superficial femoral artery are not yet available. Other devices commonly or occasionally, used in PVI, including rotational atherectomy, chronic total occlusion recanalization, and aspiration thrombectomy, are also not yet available for use via TRA.

Third, the risks of TRA for PVI for the patient and operator have not been well characterized. Among patients undergoing coronary angiography and PCI, the risk of stroke is similar in patients undergoing TRA and TFA[49]; this is likely, but not certain, to hold true in PVI. Furthermore,

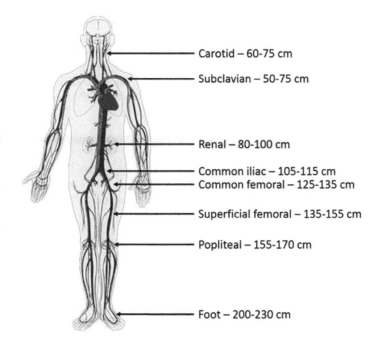

Fig. 3. Working length from left radial artery access to peripheral vascular beds. For right radial access, add 10 cm to each distance, except for carotid and subclavian artery interventions. To intervene on a lower extremity lesion via the radial approach, devices must have a working length adequate to reach and treat the lesion.

Carotid – 60-75 cm

Subclavian – 50-75 cm

Renal – 80-100 cm

Common iliac – 105-115 cm
Common femoral – 125-135 cm

Superficial femoral – 135-155 cm

Popliteal – 155-170 cm

Foot – 200-230 cm

Box 1
Technical aspects of lower extremity peripheral vascular intervention via the radial artery

A key element of lower extremity PVI via transradial access is preprocedural planning to ensure availability of devices with sufficient length to reach the lesion (see Fig. 3). Left radial access reduces the distance to the lesion and avoids instrumentation of the carotid arteries and proximal aortic arch; a left radial approach may be facilitated by abducting the patient's arm and rearranging the room so that the operator can stand on the patient's left with a scrub table arranged perpendicular to the patient to facilitate device entry and exchanges.

Radial access is obtained in the traditional manner and a short 6-Fr sheath inserted into the radial artery. Radial artery angiography is advisable to ensure a large enough artery to facilitate large-bore access. A 0.89-mm (0.035″) guidewire is then advanced into the descending thoracic artery, using a JR (Judkins right) catheter in the left anterior oblique view to direct the wire if necessary, and the 6-Fr sheath can be exchanged for a long 6-Fr guiding sheath or 7-Fr guiding catheter. These sheaths are available in 120-cm length (which can reach the common iliac arteries via radial access) and 150-cm length (which reaches the superficial femoral artery) (Terumo, Tokyo, Japan). Once the sheath is placed, the patient is anticoagulated in the traditional manner to reduce the risk of radial artery occlusion, and a wire is advanced across the lesion. Support catheters with length up to 150 cm are available.

For calcified lesions, orbital atherectomy devices with 200-cm shaft lengths are available (Cardiovascular Systems, Inc.; St Paul, MN), which reaches to the popliteal artery or beyond; 475-cm long, 0.356-cm (0.014″) wires are available for use with these devices. Two-hundred-centimeter exchange catheters are available to enable wire exchanges.

After adequate lesion preparation, rapid exchange percutaneous transluminal angioplasty balloons with 200-cm shafts that track over 0.89-mm (0.035″) wires are available with diameters ranging from 3 to 8 mm and lengths from 20 to 200 cm; balloons with 200-cm shafts that track over 0.356-mm (0.014″) wires are available with diameters ranging from 1.25 to 7 mm and lengths from 1.5 to 30 cm. Self-expanding stents are not yet available, but will be available soon, with diameters ranging from 6 to 8 mm.

When the procedure is finished, the guide catheter or sheath is withdrawn, and hemostasis is achieved using traditional radial patent hemostasis methods.

---

the mechanism explaining the lower rate of AKI with TRA compared with TFA among patients undergoing PCI is uncertain. It has been hypothesized that TRA reduces AKI both by reducing bleeding complications and by reducing atheroembolization to the renal circulation compared with TFA.[50] In contrast with coronary angiography and PCI, TRA may expose patients undergoing lower extremity PVI to a greater risk of renal artery atheroembolization than TFA,

because only TRA requires instrumentation of the abdominal aorta. In addition, in patients undergoing PCI, small studies suggest that radiation dose delivered to the patient is higher and fluoroscopy times longer with TRA compared with TFA.[51] However, the nominally higher radiation exposure with TRA is seen in low-volume centers and operators, and normalizes with TFA as procedural volumes increase.[52] This finding may also be the case for PVI, because

Table 1
Devices with shaft length and sheath size compatible for lower extremity peripheral vascular interventions via transradial access, and incompatible devices often used in peripheral intervention

	Sheath	Wire	Balloon	Drug-Coated Balloon	Stent	Covered Stent	Atherectomy	Crossing Device
Iliac	✓	✓	✓	✓	✓	✓[a]	✓ Orbital and rotational	✓
Femoral-Popliteal	✓	✓	✓	✗	Coming soon	✗	✓ Orbital only	✗
Below the Knee	✓	✓	✓	✗	Coming soon	✗	✓ Orbital only	✗

[a] Covered stents of adequate size to be used in the iliac artery require 7-Fr access.

of the early learning curve and greater procedural complexity with TRA. In the current TFA era, 1 in 14 patients undergoing PVI receives a dosage greater than 500 Gy × cm², which is the threshold for tissue injury.[53] As TRA for PVI grows, data on volume and radiation exposure will be important to analyze.

FUTURE DIRECTIONS

The development of new technology to facilitate lower extremity PVI via TRA carries promise for improved patient outcomes, primarily via a reduction in bleeding. However, there is limited experience with TRA for these procedures, and feasibility and outcomes need to be better characterized (Table 2). The National Cardiovascular Data Registry's PVI Registry collects data on arterial access; data on the uptake and procedural outcomes of TRA for PVI will be important, including rates of crossover to TFA, vascular access complications, bleeding, stroke, AKI, and radiation dose. Ultimately, as more devices are developed and TRA for PVI matures, a clinical trial randomizing patients undergoing lower extremity PVI to TRA versus TFA to determine the effect of TRA on procedural success and key outcomes, such as bleeding, stroke, and AKI, will be necessary to determine whether TRA should become standard of care for PVI.

Table 2
Benefits and concerns of transradial access (compared with transfemoral access) for peripheral vascular intervention

Potential Benefits	Concerns

• Lower risk of severe vascular access complications
  ○ Lower hospital costs?
  ○ Lower mortality?
• Lower risk of acute kidney injury related to acute blood-loss anemia
• Shorter time on bed rest
• Greater patient satisfaction
• Improved ergonomics for operator, especially for right leg interventions
• Ability to intervene on both legs during 1 procedure
	• Unknown risk of stroke and acute kidney injury
	• Limited availability of devices with adequate length
	• Higher rate of radial artery spasm in patients with PAD
	• Calcified and stenotic arm arteries may increase procedural complexity
	• Higher procedural complexity may increase patient radiation exposure
	• Limited evidence base documenting safety and efficacy

REFERENCES

1. Fowkes FGR, Rudan D, Rudan I, et al. Comparison of global estimates of prevalence and risk factors for peripheral artery disease in 2000 and 2010: a systematic review and analysis. Lancet 2013; 382(9901):1329–40.
2. Scully RE, Arnaoutakis DJ, DeBord Smith A, et al. Estimated annual health care expenditures in individuals with peripheral arterial disease. J Vasc Surg 2018;67(2):558–67.
3. Marrett E, DiBonaventura Md, Zhang Q. Burden of peripheral arterial disease in Europe and the United States: a patient survey. Health Qual Life Outcomes 2013;11(1):175.
4. Sampson UK, Fowkes FG, McDermott MM, et al. Global and regional burden of death and disability from peripheral artery disease: 21 world regions, 1990 to 2010. Glob Heart 2014;9(1):145–58.e21.
5. Criqui Michael H, Aboyans V. Epidemiology of peripheral artery disease. Circ Res 2015;116(9): 1509–26.
6. McDermott MM, Greenland P, Liu K, et al. Leg symptoms in peripheral arterial disease associated clinical characteristics and functional impairment. J Am Med Assoc 2001;286(13):1599–606.
7. Soga Y, Iida O, Takahaera M, et al. Two-year life expectancy in patients with critical limb ischemia. JACC Cardiovasc Interv 2014;7(12):1444–9.
8. Freisinger E, Lüders F, Gebauer K, et al. Peripheral arterial disease and critical limb ischaemia: still poor outcomes and lack of guideline adherence. Eur Heart J 2015;36(15):932–8.
9. Vemulapalli S, Dolor RJ, Hasselblad V, et al. Comparative effectiveness of medical therapy, supervised exercise, and revascularization for patients with intermittent claudication: a network meta-analysis. Clin Cardiol 2015;38(6): 378–86.
10. Gerhard-Herman MD, Gornik HL, Barrett C, et al. 2016 AHA/ACC Guideline on the Management of Patients With Lower Extremity Peripheral Artery Disease: A Report of the American College of Cardiology/American Heart Association Task Force on Clinical Practice Guidelines. J Am Coll Cardiol 2017;69(11):e71–126.
11. Aboyans V, Ricco JB, Bartelink MEL, et al. 2017 ESC Guidelines on the Diagnosis and Treatment of Peripheral Arterial Diseases, in collaboration with the European Society for Vascular Surgery (ESVS): Document covering atherosclerotic disease of extracranial carotid and vertebral, mesenteric, renal, upper and lower extremity arteries. Endorsed by: the European Stroke Organization (ESO)The Task Force for the Diagnosis and Treatment of Peripheral Arterial Diseases of the European Society of Cardiology (ESC) and of the European Society

for Vascular Surgery (ESVS). Eur Heart J 2018;39(9): 763–816.

12. Bypass versus angioplasty in severe ischaemia of the leg (BASIL): multicentre, randomised controlled trial. Lancet 2005;366(9501):1925–34.

13. Soden PA, Zettervall SL, Curran T, et al. Regional variation in patient selection and treatment for lower extremity vascular disease in the Vascular Quality Initiative. J Vasc Surg 2017;65(1):108–18.

14. Ortiz D, Jahangir A, Singh M, et al. Access site complications after peripheral vascular interventions. Circ Cardiovasc Interv 2014;7(6):821–8.

15. Doyle BJ, Ting HH, Bell MR, et al. Major femoral bleeding complications after percutaneous coronary intervention: incidence, predictors, and impact on long-term survival among 17,901 patients treated at the Mayo Clinic From 1994 to 2005. JACC Cardiovasc Interv 2008;1(2):202–9.

16. Doyle BJ, Rihal CS, Gastineau DA, et al. Bleeding, blood transfusion, and increased mortality after percutaneous coronary intervention: implications for contemporary practice. J Am Coll Cardiol 2009;53(22):2019–27.

17. Kolkailah AA, Alreshq RS, Muhammed AM, et al. Transradial versus transfemoral approach for diagnostic coronary angiography and percutaneous coronary intervention in people with coronary artery disease. Cochrane Database Syst Rev 2018;(4):CD012318.

18. Gurm HS, Hosman C, Share D, et al. Comparative safety of vascular closure devices and manual closure among patients having percutaneous coronary intervention. Ann Intern Med 2013;159(10): 660–6.

19. Dencker D, Pedersen F, Engstrøm T, et al. Major femoral vascular access complications after coronary diagnostic and interventional procedures: a Danish register study. Int J Cardiol 2016;202: 604–8.

20. Romaguera R, Wakabayashi K, Laynez-Carnicero A, et al. Association between bleeding severity and long-term mortality in patients experiencing vascular complications after percutaneous coronary intervention. Am J Cardiol 2012;109(1):75–81.

21. Kugelmass AD, Cohen DJ, Brown PP, et al. Hospital resources consumed in treating complications associated with percutaneous coronary interventions. Am J Cardiol 2006;97(3):322–7.

22. Seto AH, Abu-Fadel MS, Sparling JM, et al. Real-time ultrasound guidance facilitates femoral arterial access and reduces vascular complications: FAUST (Femoral Arterial Access With Ultrasound Trial). JACC Cardiovasc Interv 2010;3(7):751–8.

23. Kalish J, Eslami M, Gillespie D, et al. Routine use of ultrasound guidance in femoral arterial access for peripheral vascular intervention decreases groin hematoma rates. J Vasc Surg 2015;61(5):1231–8.

24. Lo RC, Fokkema MT, Curran T, et al. Routine use of ultrasound-guided access reduces access site-related complications after lower extremity percutaneous revascularization. J Vasc Surg 2015;61(2): 405–12.

25. Inagaki E, Farber A, Siracuse JJ, et al. Routine use of ultrasound guidance in femoral arterial access for peripheral vascular intervention decreases groin hematoma rates in high-volume surgeons. Ann Vasc Surg 2018;51:1–7.

26. Martin JL, Pratsos A, Magargee E, et al. A randomized trial comparing compression, perclose proglide™ and Angio-Seal VIP™ for arterial closure following percutaneous coronary intervention: The cap trial. Catheter Cardiovasc Interv 2008;71(1):1–5.

27. Starnes BW, O'Donnell SD, Gillespie DL, et al. Percutaneous arterial closure in peripheral vascular disease: a prospective randomized evaluation of the Perclose device. J Vasc Surg 2003; 38(2):263–71.

28. Valgimigli M, Gagnor A, Calabro P, et al. Radial versus femoral access in patients with acute coronary syndromes undergoing invasive management: a randomised multicentre trial. Lancet 2015; 385(9986):2465–76.

29. Sheikh IR, Ahmed SH, Mori N, et al. Comparison of safety and efficacy of bivalirudin versus unfractionated heparin in percutaneous peripheral intervention: a single-center experience. JACC Cardiovasc Interv 2009;2(9):871–6.

30. Andò G, Cortese B, Russo F, et al. Acute kidney injury after radial or femoral access for invasive acute coronary syndrome management: AKI-MATRIX. J Am Coll Cardiol 2017;69(21):2592–603.

31. Safley David M, Salisbury Adam C, Tsai Thomas T, et al. Abstract 10709: A risk model of acute kidney injury in patients undergoing peripheral vascular intervention: from the National Cardiovascular Data Registry Peripheral Vascular Intervention (NCDR PVI) Registry™. Circulation 2018; 138(Suppl_1):A10709.

32. Amin AP, Patterson M, House JA, et al. Costs associated with access site and same-day discharge among medicare beneficiaries undergoing percutaneous coronary intervention: an evaluation of the current percutaneous coronary intervention care pathways in the United States. JACC Cardiovasc Interv 2017;10(4):342–51.

33. Liang P, Li C, O'Donnell TFX, et al. In-hospital versus postdischarge major adverse events within 30 days following lower extremity revascularization. J Vasc Surg 2019;69(2):482–9.

34. Meertens MM, Ng E, Loh SEK, et al. Transradial approach for aortoiliac and femoropopliteal interventions: a systematic review and meta-analysis. J Endovasc Ther 2018;25(5):599–607.

35. Scheinert D, Braunlich S, Nonnast-Daniel B, et al. Transradial approach for renal artery stenting. Catheter Cardiovasc Interv 2001;54(4):442–7.

36. Galli M, Tarantino F, Mameli S, et al. Transradial approach for renal percutaneous transluminal angioplasty and stenting: a feasibility pilot study. J Invasive Cardiol 2002;14(7):386–90.

37. Alli O, Mathew V, From AM, et al. Transradial access for renal artery intervention is feasible and safe. Vasc Endovascular Surg 2011;45(8):738–42.

38. Ruzsa Z, Toth K, Jambrik Z, et al. Transradial access for renal artery intervention. Interv Med Appl Sci 2014;6(3):97–103.

39. Kedev S, Zafirovska B, Petkoska D, et al. Results of transradial subclavian artery percutaneous interventions after bilateral or single access. Am J Cardiol 2016;118(6):918–23.

40. Yu J, Korabathina R, Coppola J, et al. Transradial approach to subclavian artery stenting. J Invasive Cardiol 2010;22(5):204–6.

41. Posham R, Biederman DM, Patel RS, et al. Transradial approach for noncoronary interventions: a single-center review of safety and feasibility in the first 1,500 cases. J Vasc Interv Radiol 2016;27(2):159–66.

42. Hung ML, Lee EW, McWilliams JP, et al. A reality check in transradial access: a single-centre comparison of transradial and transfemoral access for abdominal and peripheral intervention. Eur Radiol 2019;29(1):68–74.

43. Ruzsa Z, Nemes B, Pinter L, et al. A randomised comparison of transradial and transfemoral approach for carotid artery stenting: RADCAR (RADial access for CARotid artery stenting) study. EuroIntervention 2014;10(3):381–91.

44. Jolly SS, Yusuf S, Cairns J, et al. Radial versus femoral access for coronary angiography and intervention in patients with acute coronary syndromes (RIVAL): a randomised, parallel group, multicentre trial. Lancet 2011;377(9775):1409–20.

45. Deftereos S, Giannopoulos G, Kossyvakis C, et al. Radial artery flow-mediated dilation predicts arterial spasm during transradial coronary interventions. Catheter Cardiovasc Interv 2011;77(5): 649–54.

46. Truesdell AG, Delgado GA, Blakeley SW, et al. Transradial peripheral vascular intervention: challenges and opportunities. Interv Cardiol 2015;7(1): 55–76.

47. Giannopoulos G, Raisakis K, Synetos A, et al. A predictive score of radial artery spasm in patients undergoing transradial percutaneous coronary intervention. Int J Cardiol 2015;188:76–80.

48. Patel T, Shah S, Pancholy S, et al. Working through challenges of subclavian, innominate, and aortic arch regions during transradial approach. Catheter Cardiovasc Interv 2014;84(2):224–35.

49. Ferrante G, Rao SV, Jüni P, et al. Radial versus femoral access for coronary interventions across the entire spectrum of patients with coronary artery disease: a meta-analysis of randomized trials. JACC Cardiovasc Interv 2016;9(14): 1419–34.

50. Andò G, Cortese B, Frigoli E, et al. Acute kidney injury after percutaneous coronary intervention: rationale of the AKI-MATRIX (acute kidney injury-minimizing adverse hemorrhagic events by TRansradial access site and systemic implementation of angioX) sub-study. Catheter Cardiovasc Interv 2015;86(5):950–7.

51. Sciahbasi A, Frigoli E, Sarandrea A, et al. Radiation exposure and vascular access in acute coronary syndromes: The RAD-matrix trial. J Am Coll Cardiol 2017;69(20):2530–7.

52. Jolly SS, Cairns J, Niemela K, et al. Effect of radial versus femoral access on radiation dose and the importance of procedural volume: a substudy of the multicenter randomized RIVAL trial. JACC Cardiovasc Interv 2013;6(3):258–66.

53. Goldsweig AM, Kennedy KF, Abbott JD, et al. Patient radiation dosage during lower extremity endovascular intervention. JACC Cardiovasc Interv 2019;12(5):473–80.

Using the Arm for Structural Interventions
Case Selection or Wave of the Future

Pedro A. Villablanca, MD, MSc*, Tiberio Frisoli, MD,
William O'Neill, MD, Marvin Eng, MD

KEYWORDS

• Transradial • Structural heart • Transcatheter interventions

KEY POINTS

- The transradial approach has emerged as the preferred alternative to the traditional transfemoral approach owing to the increased evidence of its safety and efficacy.
- The field of structural heart disease is rapidly evolving; however, periprocedural complications related to access site remain a major determinant of morbidity and mortality.
- The transradial approach as primary or secondary access site in structural heart interventions is feasible and safe, with fewer vascular complications and high procedural success.

The advent of percutaneous therapies for cardiovascular diseases has expanded the diagnostic and therapeutic options for these patients. The transfemoral approach (TFA) has dominated the explosive growth of invasive cardiology in past decades. Advances toward smaller sheath sizes and maturation of both devices and operator experience has helped to lower the rate of periprocedural complications; however, the TFA still contributes to periprocedural morbidity and mortality via access site complications.[1,2]

The transradial approach (TRA) has emerged as the preferred access site in coronary angiography and intervention owing to the increased evidence of its safety and efficacy.[3] Although the TRA can be more challenging with certain disadvantages compared with the TFA (eg, steep learning curve, greater radiation exposure, and limitation of therapeutic equipment), the body of evidence demonstrate a significant reduction in bleeding and vascular complications, lower associated health care costs, and improved patient satisfaction with the TRA versus the TFA.[4,5] The benefits observed in coronary interventions has expanded the use of this approach for peripheral endovascular and neurointerventional procedures with comparable results: similar efficacy and lower rates of vascular complications compared with the TFA.[6,7]

The field of structural heart disease is rapidly evolving, with major refinements in technology, procedural techniques, and patient selection. For example, transcatheter aortic valve replacement (TAVR) in appropriately selected patients is now offered as a less invasive option compared with conventional surgery. Traditionally, large-bore catheters and surgical cutdowns were used for such procedures. However, advances in frame material, leaflet design, and loading and delivery catheter systems now allow us now to deliver transcatheter valves through 14F sheaths as compared with the initial 25F sheaths. Despite these advancements, however, access site complications remain a major determinant of TAVR morbidity and mortality.[8]

The use of TRA varies among different countries and even different operators in the same center with a low prevalence in the United States.[9] In structural heart interventions, the incidence of TRA use is even lower. In this review,

Center for Structural Heart Disease, Henry Ford Hospital, 2799 West Grand Boulevard, Detroit, MI 48202, USA
* Corresponding author.
E-mail addresses: pedrovillablanca@hotmail.com; pvillab1@hfhs.org

Intervent Cardiol Clin 9 (2020) 63–74
https://doi.org/10.1016/j.iccl.2019.08.007
2211-7458/20/© 2019 Elsevier Inc. All rights reserved.

we present the feasibility and safety of TRA during structural heart disease interventions and optimal strategies to apply the TRA approach in this challenging group of patients (Fig. 1).

BALLOON AORTIC VALVULOPLASTY

The use of balloon aortic valvuloplasty (BAV) has undergone a resurgence in the age of TAVR.[10] Not only can BAV be used to assess aortic annulus diameter in conjunction with imaging modalities such as transesophageal echocardiography or computed tomography scans when there is discrepancy between modalities,[11] but also to optimize valve expansion after deployment in native or bioprosthetic valves.[12,13] However, in the current era of TAVR, the most common indications for BAV use has been as a bridge to TAVR or surgical aortic valve replacement or as a stratification tool for select high-risk patients whose symptoms may not be primarily cardiac in origin.[14,15]

BAV is most frequently performed in a retrograde fashion using the TFA. Occasionally, the TFA is a challenge owing to vascular disease with prohibitive atherosclerotic disease, tortuosity, calcification, or morbid obesity. The complication rate from this procedure is not negligible, an alternative access route may be considered.[10]

Recently transradial aortic valvuloplasty (TRAV) has been described as a minimally invasive modality to perform BAV. The use of a low-profile compliant balloon via TRA has been performed using a single 8F or 9F sheath via a right or left radial approach[16] but also via bilateral 6F radial artery access.[17] The largest series published is an early safety and feasibility study of 30 patients who underwent TRAV with rapid pacing through a 0.035-inch left ventricular support wire. TRAV was successful in all patients but one, who required a crossover to TFA because of the inability to deliver a valvuloplasty balloon through a severely calcified radial artery. There were no balloon entrapments or compartment syndromes. The mean invasive gradient across the aortic valve decreased by at least 30% in 90% of patients. At 30-day echocardiographic follow-up, the radial artery was patent in 80%, and there were no significant differences between pre- and post-TRAV handgrip strength test in the instrumented arm.[18] Based on the present pilot study, the same group has set in place a larger prospective registry (Mini-invasive Balloon Aortic Valvuloplasty; SOFTLY-II) to confirm these preliminary data (NCT03087552).

How to perform the procedure? Ultrasound guidance can be useful to address patency and size of the radial artery and determine whether it is large enough to accommodate the necessary sheath. The radial artery is much smaller, averaging 2.6 mm in diameter compared with 7 mm for the femoral artery, and calcification of the artery may cause the artery to move away from the needle tip. Ultrasound guidance improves the success and efficiency of radial artery cannulation in patients presenting for transradial catheterization[19] and decrease the number of attempts required to access the radial artery.[20,21] In addition, assessment of the size of the artery allows for estimation of the likelihood of artery occlusion after the procedure. It has been shown that when the sheath outer diameter exceeds the radial artery diameter, radial artery occlusion may be more likely.[22] Once access is obtained, local standards of each laboratory should be used to prevent radial artery occlusion and spasm.[5] Verapamil or nicardipin can be used to optimize artery dilation in anticipation of large sheath insertion followed by unfractionated heparin. Nitroglycerin should be avoided in critical aortic stenosis and unstable patients.[23,24] Venous access via the antecubital approach may be used to deliver the pacer wire, and in case of difficulties advancing the pacer wire, a long intravenous sheath may be used. An alternative option is to use the left ventricular guidewire for pacing where the cathode of an external pacemaker is placed on the tip of the 0.035-inch wire and the anode on a needle inserted at the access site; insulation is ensured by the balloon catheter.[25] Once venous and arterial access sites are achieved, heparin is administered intravenously and activated clotting times monitored to maintain at more than 200 seconds. For the unilateral TRAV approach, various low-profile semicompliant balloons have been used, including Tyshak balloons (Braun Interventional Systems, Bethlehem, PA) that range from 22 to 30 mm and require an 8F to 9F sheath, Cristal Balloon (Balt Extrusion, Montmorency, France) that is 22 mm and requires an 8F sheath, and the VACS II balloon (Osypka, Rheinfelden, Germany) that is 20 mm and requires an 8F sheath. In fact, semicompliant balloon material enables some variation of diameter above or below the nominal level. The balloon is often delivered across the aortic valve on a stiff body 0.035-inch wire with a safety curl at the left ventricular end of the wire. To minimize the risk of radial spasm or injury when using a sheath 8F or greater, the sheath may be inserted only half its length. If an 8F sheath

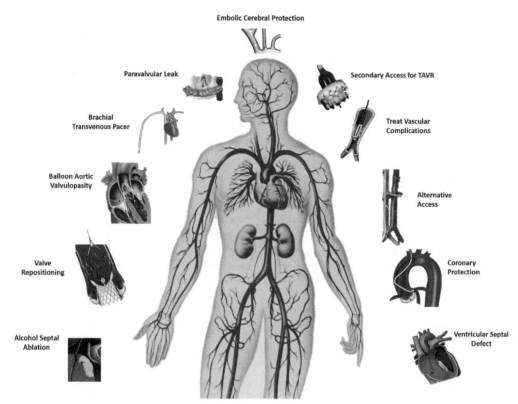

Fig. 1. Transradial/upper extremity access for structural heart interventions.

cannot be placed in the radial artery owing to a small caliber artery and the possibility of a single large sheath in the radial artery is excluded, a bilateral TRAV approach may be also considered via bilateral 6F to 7F radial artery access (Fig. 2). Two 6F or 7F sheaths are placed (one in each radial artery), depending on the balloon size

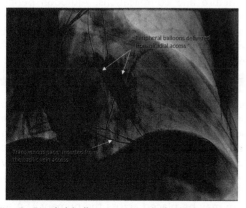

Fig. 2. Biradial balloon aortic valvuloplasty. Two peripheral Balloons 14 × 60mm and 12 × 60mm delivered over wires. A transvenous pacer was inserted from the basilic vein access to performed balloon aortic valvuloplasty.

selected. Temporary pacing can be delivered via a 5F to 6F sheath in the internal jugular, brachiocephalic, or femoral vein. Hemodynamic monitoring can be obtained using a 4F left femoral arterial access or when feasible just use a 7F radial sheath and an angioplasty balloons that would not be occlusive so pressure can be transduce from the side port (this will depend on the anatomic annular dimensions that will define which balloon size will be required). Valve hemodynamics and crossing can be performed with standard catheters and 260-cm exchange wires across the aortic valve. Two independent pressure insufflators can be used for each balloon or the balloons can be connected to a male-to-male connector, which will require one pressure insufflators. The determination of the peripheral balloon sizing is based on annular dimensions; that is, if the annular diameter is 24 mm, two 12 × 60 mm Armada balloons (Abbott Vascular, Santa Clara, CA) can be used. Finally, if a radial access sheath is a concern owing to small vessel caliber and femoral access cannot be used, an antegrade transseptal approach with externalization of a stiff guidewire as a rail via the radial artery could be an alternative. After transseptal puncture, a

7F wedge catheter can be delivered into the left ventricle and across the aortic valve. Then insert a 0.032-inch soft guide wire, and the tip of the guide wire advance into the brachial artery and exchanged for a stiff guide wire. The tip of the stiff guide wire can be externalized from the radial artery.[26] However, this approach has a non-negligible rate of access-related and non–access-related complications (iatrogenic atrial septal defect and cardiac tamponade) and should be done by trained or experience operators.

The ultimate question will be if TRAV is overall a safer bridge to surgery or TAVR than the TFA approach when feasible. Although technological advances in arterial device delivery systems have diminished the risk of procedural access complications, access complications still exist in patients with severe calcified stenosis and other anatomic reasons for non-navigability of current catheter delivery systems. Furthermore, we should recognize that the available balloons for TRA have lower profiles but also burst at lower pressures. Improvements in the size, compliance, burst pressure, profile, and cone angle of balloon catheters will be pivotal in continuing to improve TRAV technology. But among these characteristics, profile is perhaps the most important. Randomized studies are warranted to establish the potential safety and effectiveness of TRAV compared with BAV via TFA.

TRANSCATHETER AORTIC VALVE IMPLANTATION

A significant component of the morbidity and mortality of TAVR has been associated with major vascular complications.[27,28] The risk of vascular trauma increases with larger sheath sizes, and the development of lower profile TAVR delivery systems has shown a decrease in vascular complication rates.[29] Although rates have improved, they are still not and the effective management of vascular access complications is of paramount importance because the pool of potential TAVR candidates is likely to increase given the recent data demonstrating noninferiority with TAVR versus surgical aortic valve replacement in low-risk patients.[30,31]

All of the approved commercially available valves in the United States required a secondary access to complete the TAVR procedure. This secondary access is used (1) for placement of a pigtail catheter in the aortic root to define the annular plane, (2) to perform aortography to aid valve positioning and embolic protection deployment, (3) to assess for potential procedural complications, (4) to guide the puncture for primary femoral arterial access, (5) to identify vascular complications at the site of the large-bore sheath and ensure adequate hemostasis, and (6) in the event of vascular complications, secondary arterial access can be used to perform peripheral intervention. All of these tasks can be accomplished with the TRA.

Although most operators use the contralateral femoral artery as the secondary arterial access for TAVR, several recent nonrandomized studies have investigated the outcomes of the TRA as secondary access in TAVR with promising results.[32–35] A report by Allende and colleagues[33] evaluated the use of TRA versus TFA as secondary access during TAVR in 462 patients (TRA in 127 patients vs TFA in 335 patients). The use of the TRA as a secondary access site was associated with a lower rate of vascular complications (0% vs 5.0%; $P = .014$) and major and/or life-threatening bleeding events related to the secondary access site (0% vs 3%; $P = .049$) when compared with the TFA. Subsequent studies have demonstrated similar results.[32,34,35] The crossover rate from s TRA to a TFA is low (<3%), which is an acceptable rate considering the vascular tortuosity in the TAVR population.[32] Furthermore, use of a TRA over a TFA as the secondary access site is not associated with an increase in procedural time or amount of contrast used. However, a higher procedural fluoroscopy time has been observed with TRA when compared with the TFA.[35]

The TRA may not only decrease vascular complications at the secondary access site, but also be effective at managing primary access site puncture and complications. Although peripheral angiography and intervention may be more challenging via TRA because the majority of equipment is designed for use from a TFA, many times a secondary TFA access site is not feasible or may prove challenging in diffusely diseased and excessively tortuous vessels with narrow iliac bifurcations angles. With the appropriate equipment developed for TRA intervention, most peripheral vascular complications can be managed entirely via TRA.[36,37] One retrospective cohort of patients undergoing a TFA TAVR report demonstrated that usage of the TRA as the secondary access site via which a wire may be placed across the primary TFA access site for accurate TFA puncture is safe with no difference in major or minor vascular complications (8.7% vs 9.8%, $P = .86$) and numerically fewer life-threatening (9.1% vs 19.5%; $P = .17$)

and major bleeding events (13.6% vs 22%; P = .32) observed in the TRA versus the TFA for secondary access group.[38] In a more recent cohort, Jackson and colleagues[34] used the TRA as secondary access in 64% of the TAVR cases. In the TRA cohort, percutaneous vascular intervention was performed from the TRA in 17%, and emergent secondary TFA access was not required in any case. There are lines of peripheral balloons available with 150-, 170-, and 180-cm shaft lengths that are compatible with an 0.014-inch and 0.018-inch wire and a 6F guide. Nitinol self-expanding stents are also available with a 180-cm shaft length that can be delivered by a 6F catheter. However, there are, unfortunately, currently no covered stents with long enough shaft lengths to be deployed in the common femoral artery via the TRA.

ALTERNATIVE ACCESS FOR TRANSCATHETER AORTIC VALVE REPLACEMENT

With lower profile TAVR delivery systems,[39] the need for alternative surgical access has declined over time. However, there remain a number of patients who are not candidates for TAVR via the TFA given that the prevalence of peripheral arterial vascular disease in this patient population is about 25%.[40] Therefore, when TAVR cannot be performed via the TFA, it is important for the valve team to be knowledgeable in alternative access approaches (subclavian/axillary, transcarotid, transcaval) and safe closure.

For subclavian access, the role of the TRA plays a key role as the secondary arterial access site during dilation and sheath delivery. When the left subclavian artery approach is used, some operators prefer the TFA as a secondary access site and externalize an 0.018-inch wire

out the left radial artery as a third arterial access. However, one may choose to have only 2 arterial access sites with a peripheral over-the-wire balloon (shaft length of ≥130 cm) sized 1:1 with the subclavian artery delivered from the left radial artery using either a 6F or 7F thin-walled sheath and with the wire positioned in the proximal or midportion of the descending aorta. The peripheral balloon can be inflated between device exchanges to minimize blood loss by inflating to 1 to 2 atm as equipment is removed from the arteriotomy. At our center, when subclavian access is considered, the preference is to use a 7F sheath and an over-the-wire peripheral balloon with an 0.035-inch lumen to avoid loss of wire position. This method allows us to perform angiography of the vessel while the balloon and wire are still in place, and also allows for delivery of a covered stent if needed without a need to upsize the sheath or obtain another access. The temporary pacemaker can be delivered either from the internal jugular or brachiocephalic vein (**Fig. 3**).

Transcaval access is offered to patients who are not eligible for TFA access and who do not have good alternative arterial access options. Planning includes a preprocedure contrast-enhanced computed tomography scan of the abdomen and pelvis. Typically, arterial access is necessary for aortography, snaring and tensioning the transcaval guidewire, and TAVR-related aortography.[41] Most frequently, TFA is used to perform this maneuver. Given that the length of snares is not enough to reach the infrarenal descending aorta from the TRA, the operator can consider a 6F sheath via the brachial artery as the second arterial access during transcaval TAVR (**Fig. 4**). Depending on the size of the abdominal aorta, a bailout strategy for endovascular aortic stenting will require the

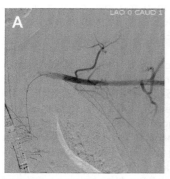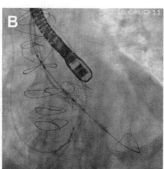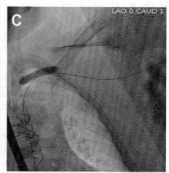

Fig. 3. Bilateral subclavian and radial access for TAVR. (*A*) Externalization of glide wire from left to right TRA and a peripheral balloon advanced for dry access of the left subclavian artery. (*B*) TAVR valve deployed from left subclavian artery, a pigtail from right TRA for aortogram, and a transvenous pacer from right internal jugular. (*C*) Peripheral balloon from right TRA inflated for dry closure of the TAVR sheath access.

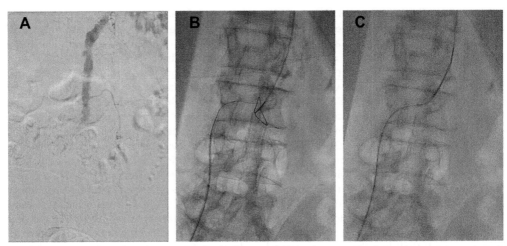

Fig. 4. Transcaval access technique for TAVR using the left brachial artery. (*A*) Aortogram showing occluded left and right common iliac arteries. (*B*) Transcaval access is obtained over an electrified guidewire directed from the inferior vena cava toward a snare delivered from the left brachial artery to the abdominal aorta. (*C*) The 0.014-inch guidewire was snared successfully and is ready to be advanced to the aortic arch.

brachial sheath to be upsized to a 7F or 8F sheath or subclavian artery access may need to be considered to facilitate delivery of equipment.

Transcarotid access offers direct vascular access to the aortic valve. Like the alternative accesses discussed elsewhere in this article, the indications for a transcarotid approach include patients who cannot tolerate a TFA and who also have an absolute or relative contraindication to a direct aortic approach. This approach for TAVR is safe and feasible and is associated with encouraging short-term clinical outcomes compared with the more invasive transapical or transaortic strategies.[42] Much like the exposure for a carotid endarterectomy, proximal and distal control is obtained and the artery is accessed with a 5F sheath. The valve is then crossed and the carotid artery dilated to accommodate a 14F to 16F sheath for device delivery and deployment. The secondary TRA can be used either from the left or right radial artery. The secondary access in this scenario is mainly to define placement of the pigtail catheter in the aortic root and to perform aortography to aid valve positioning and ensure adequate hemostasis at the access site that is surgically closed. Vascular complications are usually treated surgically; however, the right radial artery could be used for possible endovascular interventions, if needed, into the right carotid or left carotid in case of bovine arch. A TRA for nonbovine left internal carotid disease is more challenging owing to the unfavorable takeoff of the left common carotid.[43] A 5F or 6F guiding

sheath would be required to deliver a stent. The temporary pacemaker can be delivered either from the contralateral internal jugular or either brachiocephalic vein.

TRANSCATHETER AORTIC VALVE REPLACEMENT REPOSITIONING

The new Medtronic transcatheter heart valve CoreValve Evolut Pro system (Medtronic, Inc., Minneapolis, MN) offers many advantages, including the ability to recapture and reposition the bioprosthesis at deployments of up to 80%.[44] However, once these valves are fully deployed, the only way to reposition or retrieve these valves after attempting other maneuvers to mitigate the aortic insufficiency (ie, post dilatation) is to snare it back.[45,46] This technique may be applied when the aortic prosthesis is initially positioned too low, causing significant aortic insufficiency or too high causing coronary obstruction. For the first scenario, snaring and repositioning the valve should be performed with caution owing to the risk of embolization, but also, when the valve is pulled back, there is a risk of coronary obstruction with the valve's skirt; in this event, the valve should be pulled back even more. In the scenario of coronary obstruction (especially in valve-in-valve procedures), snaring of the valve should be perform immediately as another operator is trying to regain access of the left coronary ostium. For this emergency, the operator needs 2 secondary access points: one to snare the valve and the second to cannulate the coronary artery; either the TRA or the TFA can be used for any of those task. More often, the TFA is used to cannulate the coronary artery, and the TRA would be the most expeditious if it is the only access available to snare it (**Fig. 5**). Frequently, a second snare is needed to pull the inner tab while the first snare pulls the outer tab; in that case, the snaring can be performed using both radial arteries. Snaring via the TRA can be performed using a 6F sheath. We recommend an EN Snare Device (Merit Medical System, South Jordan, UT) that has 3 interlaced loops designed to rotate and expand for excellent coverage and retrieval. The snare can be directed through a 6F JR4 guiding catheter.

EMBOLIC PROTECTION DEVICE

Several adverse events are associated with TAVR, prime among them being cerebrovascular events. During the early phases of TAVR, the incidence of stroke was up to 10%, but in the latest studies and meta-analyses, the incidence of stroke has decreased to rates comparable with those with surgical aortic valve replacement at close to 3%.[47] Cerebral embolic protection devices have been developed to minimize the risk of periprocedural ischemic stroke during TAVR. Several randomized controlled trials have evaluated the safety and efficacy of cerebral embolic protection devices in TAVR with a nonsignificant decrease in new lesion volume on magnetic resonance scans.[48,49] Nonetheless, a recent meta-analysis of cerebral embolic protection devices demonstrated a decreased incidence of strokes within 1 week of follow-up without showing any evidence of increased risk of other periprocedural adverse events.[50]

There are currently two devices available during TAVR that can be delivered via TRA using a 6F sheath.[51] Currently, the only US Food and Drug Administration-approved device, the

Sentinel Cerebral Protection System (Boston Scientific, Marlborough, Mass), consists of a dual filter system deployed via the right radial or brachial approach to the brachiocephalic and left common carotid arteries. It consists of a proximal filter (sized 9–15 mm in diameter) delivered in the brachiocephalic artery covering all areas of the brain supplied by the right vertebral and right carotid artery and a distal filter (sized 6.5–10.0 mm in diameter) delivered in the left common carotid artery (**Fig. 6**). The left vertebral artery, which usually originates from the left subclavian artery, remains unprotected, as does the cerebral regions fed by this vessel.[52] In high-risk cases, we have used a peripheral balloon from the left radial artery to occlude the left subclavian artery while delivering and deploying the valve.

CORONARY OBSTRUCTION

Symptomatic coronary obstruction owing to the displacement of the calcified native valve leaflets over the coronary ostia is a potential complication of TAVR. Risk factors include balloon-expandable valve, previous surgical bioprosthesis, low coronary ostium, and shallow sinus of Valsalva. Despite successful treatment, acute and late mortality remain very high, highlighting the importance of anticipating and preventing the occurrence of this complication.[53]

Preprocedural planning, including computed tomography analysis, is key to analyzing the anatomic risk factors for coronary obstruction, as well as detailing the information for the surgical prosthesis for valve-in-valve procedures. If there is risk of obstruction, coronary protection can be performed with a guide extension over a guidewire positioned in the coronary artery, which is left in place during valve deployment.

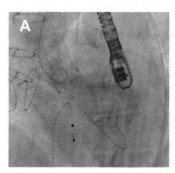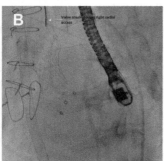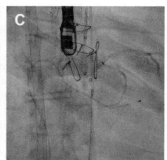

Fig. 5. Emergent valve snaring for coronary obstruction. (*A*) TAVR after deployment occluding left coronary artery. (*B*) Snaring of the valve and repositioning with EN snare device (*yellow arrow*). (*C*) Coronary guide extension over a guidewire positioned in the coronary ready to deploy a stent in the left main. ([*B*] *Courtesy of* Merit Medical System, South Jordan, UT.)

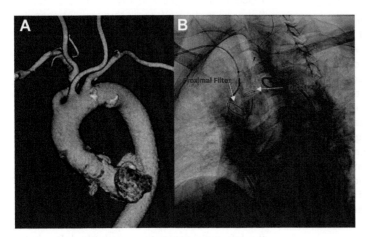

Fig. 6. Embolic protection device. (A) Preoperative 3-dimensional computed tomography reconstruction of the ascending aorta and supra-aortic vessels planning the safety and feasibility to deliver embolic protection device. (B) Sentinel Cerebral Protection System deployed from the right TRA using a 6F sheath; arrows pointing at the proximal filter in the innominate artery and the distal filter in the left common carotid. ([B] Courtesy of Boston Scientific, Inc., Marlborough, MA.)

The guide catheter is then withdrawn above the level of the leaflet insertion of the prosthetic valve, leaving the guideliner and guidewire in place, so that patency of the coronary ostia can be clearly visualized. After deployment of the valve, aortography is performed to demonstrate patency of the coronary arteries. Some operators advocate the positioning of an undeployed stent distal to the coronary ostium ready to be pulled back and deployed if necessary.[54] When TAVR is performed using the TFA as a primary access, a bilateral TRA can be used for both the traditional secondary access and coronary guide positioning. Alternatively, the potentially affected coronary arteries may be protected with intentional laceration of the bioprosthetic or native aortic scallop (BASILICA) using the contralateral TFA.[55] In cases when valve fracture is considered, the coronaries should still be protected using TRA and deferring to TFA when the BASILICA procedure is considered.

PARAVALVULAR LEAK

Percutaneous closure of a paravalvular leak (PVL) has been described as a safe and effective strategy to reduce the regurgitant volume and improve symptoms; these interventions are usually performed using the TFA.[56] The need for early restoration of anticoagulation to prevent valves thrombosis after PVL treatment in patients with mechanical valves can increase the risk of vascular complications and major bleeding. In addition, patients with mechanical valve prosthesis can also have thrombotic event owing to potential inadequate anticoagulation during periprocedural bridge therapy.[57] Although the TRA could be a limitation for bigger devices, devices are available for delivery through diagnostic catheters.[58] Hildick-Smith

and colleagues[59] reported the first case of aortic valve PVL closure using a TRA. Although the distance from the radial artery to the aortic valve may be a few centimeters shorter, a 125-mm 6F multipurpose catheter may be used inside an 8F guiding catheter as a buddy/dilator. The multipurpose catheter allows the guiding catheter to successfully cross the defect and treat the PVL with transcatheter vascular plug devices by modifying the terminal portion of the guide and facilitate engagement of the occluder sheath into the guiding catheter. If this is not an alternative, a percutaneous brachial artery approach can be used to overcome the short sheath. Two mechanical aortic valve PVL cases have been reported using a TRA with a 6F 90-cm sheath. In both cases, the PVL was sealed using a single transcatheter vascular plug.[60] Most recently, use of the TRA was reported in 2 cases of PVL closure after TAVR using a 5F sheath with a transcatheter vascular plug.[61] Last, to avoid an arteriovenous loop with a transseptal puncture, a successful closure of a TAVR PVL may be performed using the TFA and TRA for the creation of an arterio-arterial loop to gain support for advancement of the delivery sheath into the left ventricle.[62]

ALCOHOL SEPTAL ABLATION FOR HYPERTROPHIC OBSTRUCTIVE CARDIOMYOPATHY

Alcohol septal ablation (ASA) is a transcatheter approach to reduce left ventricular outflow tract gradient in patients with hypertrophic obstructive cardiomyopathy refractory to maximal medical therapy.[63,64]

ASA for treating hypertrophic obstructive cardiomyopathy was one of the first transcatheter procedures that seemed to be feasible via the

TRA, largely owing to the fact that procedural access was accomplished via 6F-compatible catheters. Cuisset and colleagues[65] reported an initial series of 30 consecutive patients successfully undergoing ASA using a complete TRA approach. Temporary pacemakers were implanted via the subclavian vein, without access site complications. After this initial successful experience, the short- and long-term (mean of 4.5 years) efficacy and feasibility of this procedure was confirmed in a larger cohort of 240 patients. The procedure success rate was 91.9% and 91.2% in the TRA and TFA groups, respectively ($P = .53$); however, vascular complications were less frequent in the TRA group (0.58% vs 7.3%; $P = .002$).[66] Although most centers used a single radial arterial access, the procedure can be performed using a minimalistic approach with a bilateral TRA with the second access site used for continuous gradient monitoring along with a right basilic vein access to place the temporary pacemaker. Most recently, ASA has emerged as a strategy to modify the left ventricular outflow tract either before or after transcatheter mitral valve replacement.[67,68] Although the initial experience was performed via the TFA, either a bilateral TRA or TRA and TFA for continuous gradient monitoring while performing the ASA may be used (Fig. 7).

VENTRICULAR SEPTAL DEFECTS

Percutaneous device closure of ventricular septal defects (VSD) has shown great success as a

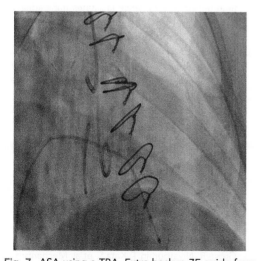

Fig. 7. ASA using a TRA. Extra backup 7F guide from the right radial was used to perform septal ablation, and the first septal artery was obliterated with an alcohol injection; Simultaneous continuous gradient monitoring with a 6F dual lumen pigtail from the left radial artery.

sustainable alternative to surgical closure.[69,70] Traditionally, the femoral artery and femoral vein or jugular vein have been used for VSD closure.[71] Data using the TRA or upper extremities are limited to a case of percutaneous closure of a perimembranous VSD via TRA and basilic vein access.[72] A 5F JR4 diagnostic catheter and an angled, torqueable 0.035-inch wire is used to cross the VSD and advance the catheter into the right ventricle. Subsequently, a guidewire is snared in the pulmonary artery via right basilic vein access. A 7F 90-cm sheath is advanced from the basilic vein, across the VSD, across the aortic valve into the right subclavian artery. Under angiographic and TEE guidance, an 8-mm VSD occlusion device may be then deployed. This innovative approach may not only offer a safer access option, but also provide a feasible alternative, particularly when access choices are limited.

LIMITATIONS OF THE TRANSRADIAL APPROACH FOR STRUCTURAL INTERVENTIONS

TRA has shown to have multiple advantages when compared with the TFA, including fewer vascular complications, reduced morbidity, decreased length of stay, early ambulation, reduced cost, and improved clinical outcomes. However, there remain several limitations of TRA for structural interventions. First, there is a limited range of interventional equipment available of sufficient length and size to be delivered via TRA for structural interventions. In addition, bailout equipment is limited; balloons and stents with long (ideally 180 cm) catheter shafts are required to reach the common femoral artery or distal vessels. Nonetheless, 150-cm catheters reach the common femoral artery in most patients. Second, vessel tortuosity may make equipment delivery difficult. In cases felt to be at high risk for vascular complications, we ensure that access to the peripheral vasculature is possible by passing a pigtail or multipurpose catheter around the arch and into the descending aorta before sheath removal. This situation can usually be managed, but occasionally does require conversion to a TFA. Third, the challenges associated with the TRA and low uptake of this technology may be partly related to technical proficiency for new operators. The concept of a learning curve, in which operator skill improves with greater experience, has been observed for many procedures, including the TRA.[73] Fourth, only case reports and observational series are available for structural radial interventions as compared with the TFA, with a big gap in evidence assessing efficacy and safety of the approach.

REFERENCES

1. Agostoni P, Biondi-Zoccai GG, de Benedictis ML, et al. Radial versus femoral approach for percutaneous coronary diagnostic and interventional procedures; Systematic overview and meta-analysis of randomized trials. J Am Coll Cardiol 2004;44(2):349–56.

2. Karrowni W, Vyas A, Giacomino B, et al. Radial versus femoral access for primary percutaneous interventions in ST-segment elevation myocardial infarction patients: a meta-analysis of randomized controlled trials. JACC Cardiovasc Interv 2013;6(8):814–23.

3. Kolkailah AA, Alreshq RS, Muhammed AM, et al. Transradial versus transfemoral approach for diagnostic coronary angiography and percutaneous coronary intervention in people with coronary artery disease. Cochrane Database Syst Rev 2018;(4):CD012318.

4. Rao SV, Cohen MG, Kandzari DE, et al. The transradial approach to percutaneous coronary intervention: historical perspective, current concepts, and future directions. J Am Coll Cardiol 2010;55(20):2187–95.

5. Mason PJ, Shah B, Tamis-Holland JE, et al. An update on radial artery access and best practices for transradial coronary angiography and intervention in acute coronary syndrome: a scientific statement from the American Heart Association. Circ Cardiovasc Interv 2018;11(9):e000035.

6. Kumar AJ, Jones LE, Kollmeyer KR, et al. Radial artery access for peripheral endovascular procedures. J Vasc Surg 2017;66(3):820–5.

7. Chen SH, Snelling BM, Shah SS, et al. Transradial approach for flow diversion treatment of cerebral aneurysms: a multicenter study. J Neurointerv Surg 2019;11(8):796–800.

8. Walther T, Hamm CW, Schuler G, et al. Perioperative results and complications in 15,964 transcatheter aortic valve replacements: prospective data from the GARY Registry. J Am Coll Cardiol 2015;65(20):2173–80.

9. Feldman DN, Swaminathan RV, Kaltenbach LA, et al. Adoption of radial access and comparison of outcomes to femoral access in percutaneous coronary intervention: an updated report from the national cardiovascular data registry (2007-2012). Circulation 2013;127(23):2295–306.

10. Keeble TR, Khokhar A, Akhtar MM, et al. Percutaneous balloon aortic valvuloplasty in the era of transcatheter aortic valve implantation: a narrative review. Open Heart 2016;3(2):e000421.

11. Babaliaros VC, Junagadhwalla Z, Lerakis S, et al. Use of balloon aortic valvuloplasty to size the aortic annulus before implantation of a balloon-expandable transcatheter heart valve. JACC Cardiovasc Interv 2010;3(1):114–8.

12. Harrison JK, Hughes GC, Reardon MJ, et al. Balloon Post-dilation following implantation of a self-expanding transcatheter aortic valve bioprosthesis. JACC Cardiovasc Interv 2017;10(2):168–75.

13. Allen KB, Chhatriwalla AK, Cohen DJ, et al. Bioprosthetic valve fracture to facilitate transcatheter valve-in-valve implantation. Ann Thorac Surg 2017;104(5):1501–8.

14. Moretti C, Chandran S, Vervueren PL, et al. Outcomes of patients undergoing balloon aortic valvuloplasty in the TAVI era: a multicenter registry. J Invasive Cardiol 2015;27(12):547–53.

15. Arsalan M, Khan S, Golman J, et al. Balloon aortic valvuloplasty to improve candidacy of patients evaluated for transcatheter aortic valve replacement. J Interv Cardiol 2018;31(1):68–73.

16. Rau EM, El-Hajjar M. Aortic valvuloplasty via the radial artery: case reports and review of the literature. Catheter Cardiovasc Interv 2018;92(3):597–600.

17. Samuel R, Hiew C, Mok M. Balloon aortic valvuloplasty via a bilateral trans-radial artery approach prior to transcatheter aortic valve replacement. J Card Surg 2018;33(10):604–6.

18. Tumscitz C, Campo G, Tebaldi M, et al. Safety and feasibility of transradial mini-invasive balloon aortic valvuloplasty: a pilot study. JACC Cardiovasc Interv 2017;10(13):1375–7.

19. Seto AH, Roberts JS, Abu-Fadel MS, et al. Real-time ultrasound guidance facilitates transradial access: RAUST (Radial Artery access with Ultrasound Trial). JACC Cardiovasc Interv 2015;8(2):283–91.

20. Shiloh AL, Savel RH, Paulin LM, et al. Ultrasound-guided catheterization of the radial artery: a systematic review and meta-analysis of randomized controlled trials. Chest 2011;139(3):524–9.

21. Moussa Pacha H, Alahdab F, Al-Khadra Y, et al. Ultrasound-guided versus palpation-guided radial artery catheterization in adult population: a systematic review and meta-analysis of randomized controlled trials. Am Heart J 2018;204:1–8.

22. Saito S, Ikei H, Hosokawa G, et al. Influence of the ratio between radial artery inner diameter and sheath outer diameter on radial artery flow after transradial coronary intervention. Catheter Cardiovasc Interv 1999;46(2):173–8.

23. Grose R, Nivatpumin T, Katz S, et al. Mechanism of nitroglycerin effect in valvular aortic stenosis. Am J Cardiol 1979;44(7):1371–7.

24. Tebbe U, Neuhaus KL, Sauer G, et al. Nitrates in aortic valve disease: acute and chronic effects. Z Kardiol 1983;72(Suppl 3):152–5.

25. Faurie B, Abdellaoui M, Wautot F, et al. Rapid pacing using the left ventricular guidewire: reviving an old technique to simplify BAV and TAVI procedures. Catheter Cardiovasc Interv 2016;88(6):988–93.

26. Kato H, Kubota S, Goto T, et al. Externalization of a stiff guide wire via the radial artery: a new technique to facilitate advancement of an Inoue balloon across the aortic valve in patients with aortic stenosis undergoing antegrade balloon aortic valvuloplasty. Cardiovasc Interv Ther 2016;31(2):140–6.

27. Ducrocq G, Francis F, Serfaty JM, et al. Vascular complications of transfemoral aortic valve implantation with the Edwards SAPIEN prosthesis: incidence and impact on outcome. EuroIntervention 2010;5(6):666–72.

28. Holmes DR Jr, Nishimura RA, Grover FL, et al. Annual outcomes with transcatheter valve therapy: from the STS/ACC TVT Registry. Ann Thorac Surg 2016;101(2):789–800.

29. Barbanti M, Binder RK, Freeman M, et al. Impact of low-profile sheaths on vascular complications during transfemoral transcatheter aortic valve replacement. EuroIntervention 2013;9(8):929–35.

30. Mack MJ, Leon MB, Thourani VH, et al. Transcatheter aortic-valve replacement with a balloon-expandable valve in low-risk patients. N Engl J Med 2019;380(18):1695–705.

31. Popma JJ, Deeb GM, Yakubov SJ, et al. Transcatheter aortic-valve replacement with a self-expanding valve in low-risk patients. N Engl J Med 2019;380(18):1706–15.

32. Wynne DG, Rampat R, Trivedi U, et al. Transradial secondary arterial access for transcatheter aortic valve implantation: experience and limitations. Heart Lung Circ 2015;24(7):682–5.

33. Allende R, Urena M, Cordoba JG, et al. Impact of the use of transradial versus transfemoral approach as secondary access in transcatheter aortic valve implantation procedures. Am J Cardiol 2014;114(11):1729–34.

34. Jackson MWP, Muir DF, de Belder MA, et al. Transradial secondary access to guide valve implantation and manage peripheral vascular complications during transcatheter aortic valve implantation. Heart Lung Circ 2019;28(4):637–46.

35. Fernandez-Lopez L, Chevalier B, Lefevre T, et al. Implementation of the transradial approach as an alternative vascular access for transcatheter aortic valve replacement guidance: experience from a high-volume center. Catheter Cardiovasc Interv 2019;93(7):1367–73.

36. Lorenzoni R, Lisi C, Lazzari M, et al. Tools & techniques: above the knee angioplasty by transradial access. EuroIntervention 2012;7(9):1118–9.

37. Cortese B, Trani C, Lorenzoni R, et al. Safety and feasibility of iliac endovascular interventions with a radial approach. Results from a multicenter study coordinated by the Italian Radial Force. Int J Cardiol 2014;175(2):280–4.

38. Curran H, Chieffo A, Buchanan GL, et al. A comparison of the femoral and radial crossover techniques for vascular access management in transcatheter aortic valve implantation: the Milan experience. Catheter Cardiovasc Interv 2014;83(1):156–61.

39. Toggweiler S, Leipsic J, Binder RK, et al. Management of vascular access in transcatheter aortic valve replacement: part 2: vascular complications. JACC Cardiovasc Interv 2013;6(8):767–76.

40. Mohananey D, Villablanca P, Gupta T, et al. Association of peripheral artery disease with in-hospital outcomes after endovascular transcatheter aortic valve replacement. Catheter Cardiovasc Interv 2019;94(2):249–55.

41. Lederman RJ, Babaliaros VC, Greenbaum AB. How to perform transcaval access and closure for transcatheter aortic valve implantation. Catheter Cardiovasc Interv 2015;86(7):1242–54.

42. Chamandi C, Abi-Akar R, Rodes-Cabau J, et al. Transcarotid compared with other alternative access routes for transcatheter aortic valve replacement. Circ Cardiovasc Interv 2018;11(11):e006388.

43. Etxegoien N, Rhyne D, Kedev S, et al. The transradial approach for carotid artery stenting. Catheter Cardiovasc Interv 2012;80(7):1081–7.

44. Medtronic. Evolut TAVR platform. Available at: http://www.medtronic.com/us-en/healthcare-professionals/products/cardiovascular/heart-valves-transcatheter/transcatheter-aortic-valve-replacement-platform.html. Accessed May 25, 2019.

45. Vavuranakis M, Vrachatis D, Stefanadis C. CoreValve aortic bioprosthesis: repositioning techniques. JACC Cardiovasc Interv 2010;3(5):565 [author reply: 565–6].

46. Beute TJ, Nolan MA, Merhi WM, et al. Use of EN Snare device for successful repositioning of the newest self-expanding transcatheter heart valve. SAGE Open Med Case Rep 2018;6. 2050313X18819933.

47. Davlouros PA, Mplani VC, Koniari I, et al. Transcatheter aortic valve replacement and stroke: a comprehensive review. J Geriatr Cardiol 2018;15(1):95–104.

48. Haussig S, Mangner N, Dwyer MG, et al. Effect of a cerebral protection device on brain lesions following transcatheter aortic valve implantation in patients with severe aortic stenosis: the CLEAN-TAVI randomized clinical trial. JAMA 2016;316(6):592–601.

49. Kapadia SR, Kodali S, Makkar R, et al. Protection against cerebral embolism during transcatheter aortic valve replacement. J Am Coll Cardiol 2017;69(4):367–77.

50. Mohananey D, Sankaramangalam K, Kumar A, et al. Safety and efficacy of cerebral protection devices in transcatheter aortic valve replacement: a clinical end-points meta-analysis. Cardiovasc Revasc Med 2018;19(7 Pt A):785–91.

51. Demir OM, Iannopollo G, Mangieri A, et al. The role of cerebral embolic protection devices during transcatheter aortic valve replacement. Front Cardiovasc Med 2018;5:150.

52. Food and Drug Administration Sentinel Cerebral Protection System. Available at: https://www.fda.gov/downloads/AdvisoryCommittees/Committees MeetingMaterials/MedicalDevices/MedicalDevices AdvisoryCommittee/CirculatorySystemDevicesPanel/ UCM542419.pdf. Accessed May 20, 2019.

53. Ribeiro HB, Webb JG, Makkar RR, et al. Predictive factors, management, and clinical outcomes of coronary obstruction following transcatheter aortic valve implantation: insights from a large multicenter registry. J Am Coll Cardiol 2013;62(17):1552–62.

54. Dvir D, Leipsic J, Blanke P, et al. Coronary obstruction in transcatheter aortic valve-in-valve implantation: preprocedural evaluation, device selection, protection, and treatment. Circ Cardiovasc Interv 2015;8(1) [pii:e002079].

55. Khan JM, Dvir D, Greenbaum AB, et al. Transcatheter laceration of aortic leaflets to prevent coronary obstruction during transcatheter aortic valve replacement: concept to first-in-human. JACC Cardiovasc Interv 2018;11(7):677–89.

56. Webb JG, Pate GE, Munt BI. Percutaneous closure of an aortic prosthetic paravalvular leak with an Amplatzer duct occluder. Catheter Cardiovasc Interv 2005;65(1):69–72.

57. Sanaani A, Yandrapalli S, Harburger JM. Antithrombotic management of patients with prosthetic heart valves. Cardiol Rev 2018;26(4):177–86.

58. Gafoor S, Franke J, Piayda K, et al. Paravalvular leak closure after transcatheter aortic valve replacement with a self-expanding prosthesis. Catheter Cardiovasc Interv 2014;84(1):147–54.

59. Hildick-Smith D, Behan MW, De Giovanni J. Percutaneous closure of an aortic paravalvular leak via the transradial approach. Catheter Cardiovasc Interv 2007;69(5):708–10.

60. Giacchi G, Freixa X, Hernandez-Enriquez M, et al. Minimally invasive transradial percutaneous closure of aortic paravalvular leaks: following the steps of percutaneous coronary intervention. Can J Cardiol 2016;32(12):1575.e17-9.

61. Ortega-Paz L, Regueiro A, Perdomo J, et al. Minimally invasive transradial percutaneous closure of an aortic paravalvular leaks after transcatheter aortic valve replacement. Can J Cardiol 2019;35(7):941.e1-2.

62. Estevez-Loureiro R, Benito-Gonzalez T, Gualis J, et al. Percutaneous paravalvular leak closure after CoreValve transcatheter aortic valve implantation using an arterio-arterial loop. J Thorac Dis 2017;9(2):E103–8.

63. Sorajja P, Ommen SR, Holmes DR Jr, et al. Survival after alcohol septal ablation for obstructive hypertrophic cardiomyopathy. Circulation 2012;126(20):2374–80.

64. Seggewiss H, Rigopoulos A, Welge D, et al. Long-term follow-up after percutaneous septal ablation in hypertrophic obstructive cardiomyopathy. Clin Res Cardiol 2007;96(12):856–63.

65. Cuisset T, Franceschi F, Prevot S, et al. Transradial approach and subclavian wired temporary pacemaker to increase safety of alcohol septal ablation for treatment of obstructive hypertrophic cardiomyopathy: the TRASA trial. Arch Cardiovasc Dis 2011;104(8–9):444–9.

66. Sawaya FJ, Louvard Y, Spaziano M, et al. Short and long-term outcomes of alcohol septal ablation with the trans-radial versus the trans-femoral approach: a single center-experience. Int J Cardiol 2016;220:7–13.

67. Guerrero M, Wang DD, Himbert D, et al. Short-term results of alcohol septal ablation as a bail-out strategy to treat severe left ventricular outflow tract obstruction after transcatheter mitral valve replacement in patients with severe mitral annular calcification. Catheter Cardiovasc Interv 2017;90(7):1220–6.

68. Sayah N, Urena M, Brochet E, et al. Alcohol septal ablation preceding transcatheter valve implantation to prevent left ventricular outflow tract obstruction. EuroIntervention 2018;13(17):2012–3.

69. Hijazi ZM, Hakim F, Haweleh AA, et al. Catheter closure of perimembranous ventricular septal defects using the new Amplatzer membranous VSD occluder: initial clinical experience. Catheter Cardiovasc Interv 2002;56(4):508–15.

70. Ibanez B, James S, Agewall S, et al. 2017 ESC Guidelines for the management of acute myocardial infarction in patients presenting with ST-segment elevation. Rev Esp Cardiol (Engl Ed) 2017;70(12):1082.

71. Faccini A, Butera G. Techniques, timing, and prognosis of transcatheter post myocardial infarction ventricular septal defect repair. Curr Cardiol Rep 2019;21(7):59.

72. Sanghvi K, Selvaraj N, Luft U. Percutaneous closure of a perimembranous ventricular septal defect through arm approach (radial artery and basilic vein). J Interv Cardiol 2014;27(2):199–203.

73. Hess CN, Peterson ED, Neely ML, et al. The learning curve for transradial percutaneous coronary intervention among operators in the United States: a study from the National Cardiovascular Data Registry. Circulation 2014;129(22):2277–86.

The Neuro Radialist

Pratit Patel, MD[a], Diogo C. Haussen, MD[b,c,d], Raul G. Nogueira, MD[b,c,d],
Priyank Khandelwal, MD[a,*]

KEYWORDS

- Trans-radial cerebral angiography • Distal radial access
- Distal radial approach cerebral angiography • Trans-radial neurointervention
- Artery to sheath ratio • Trans-radial mechanical thrombectomy
- Trans-radial aneurysm treatment

KEY POINTS

- Advantages of trans-radial approach for cerebral angiography.
- Appropriate patient selection.
- Technique: room setup, cannulation, vessel catheterization, interventions and closure.
- Limitations of trans-radial approach for cerebral angiography.

 Video content accompanies this article at http://www.interventional.theclinics.com.

INTRODUCTION

Trans-femoral access (TFA) has been the mainstay for cerebral angiography in practice and training for decades. However, TFA can lead to potentially life-threatening complications, which has sparked interest in trans-radial access (TRA) as a safer access option. TRA was first described in 1948 by Radner,[1] through a radial artery cutdown approach. Percutaneous radial access was described by Campeau[2] in 1989 for coronary angiography in 100 patients. Since then, a growing body of evidence supports that TRA is safer and cost-effective for patients. In contemporary times, TRA has become the first-line approach in coronary angiography. Matsumoto and colleagues[3] described TRA for neurointervention procedures in 2000. In spite of few large series showing safety and feasibility of the TRA for neurovascular procedures,[4–7] its adoption has been slow in the neuroendovascular field, although there is increasing enthusiasm. In this review, we discuss patient selection, technical details, advantages, and limitations of cerebral angiography via TRA.

ADVANTAGES

The benefits of TRA (summarized in **Box 1**) over TFA have been shown by large randomized

---

Disclosure Statement: P. Patel: The author has nothing to disclose. D.C. Haussen: Consultant for Stryker and Vesalio, Viz-AI (stock options). R.G. Nogueira: Principal Investigator, Stryker Neurovascular (DAWN trial [no compensation], Trevo2 trial), Cerenovus/Neuravi (ENDOLOW trial, no compensation); consultant to Stryker Neurovascular; steering committee member, Stryker Neurovascular (no compensation), Medtronic (SWIFT trial, SWIFT Prime trial [no compensation]), Cerenovus/Neuravi (ARISE2 trial, no compensation); angiographic core lab, Medtronic (STAR trial); executive committee member, Penumbra(no compensation); physician advisory board, Cerenovus/Neuravi, Phenox, Anaconda, Genentech, Biogen, Prolong Pharmaceuticals, Allm Inc (no compensation), Viz-AI; stock options. P. Khandelwal: The author has nothing to disclose.

[a] Department of Neurosurgery, Rutgers University, 90 Bergen Street, Suite 8100, Newark, NJ 07103, USA; [b] Department of Neurology, Emory University School of Medicine, Grady Memorial Hospital, Marcus Stroke and Neuroscience Center, 80 Jesse Hill Jr Drive SE, Box 036, Atlanta, GA 30303, USA; [c] Department of Neurosurgery, Emory University School of Medicine, Grady Memorial Hospital, Marcus Stroke and Neuroscience Center, 80 Jesse Hill Jr Drive SE, Box 036, Atlanta, GA 30303, USA; [d] Department of Radiology, Emory University School of Medicine, Grady Memorial Hospital, Marcus Stroke and Neuroscience Center, 80 Jesse Hill Jr Drive SE, Box 036, Atlanta, GA 30303, USA
* Corresponding author.
E-mail address: pk544@njms.rutgers.edu

- Minimal risk of major and minor bleeding
- Superficial location and no nearby other important anatomic structure
- Patient satisfaction due to early ambulation postprocedurally and less incidence of prolonged pain
- Reduced cost due to shorter length of stay
- Advantageous route in patients with severe obesity, pregnancy, difficult arch anatomy (eg, type III, Bovine)
- Can provide second access site when dual access is needed

clinical trials in the cardiac literature.[8,9] There is up to 73% relative reduction in major bleeding when compared with the TFA.[10] There is evidence of lower rates of minor bleeding as well as a reduced need for blood transfusion.[9] There is also a significant lower chance of developing a major vascular complication such as a large hematoma, pseudo-aneurysm, or retroperitoneal hematoma, which can result in severe morbidity or mortality.[9] The superficial position of the distal radial artery (RA) makes it easier to puncture and compress after sheath removal, and as a result there is a much lower probability of having major bleeding or vascular complication with TRA. This has translated to improved outcomes in higher risk cardiovascular patients.[10,11] Furthermore, there is an additional benefit of reduced duration of stay and procedural cost in the cardiac literature.[12,13]

Although there are no controlled studies in the cerebrovascular field comparing TRA versus TFA, many of these access site benefits may also apply in the neurosciences. There are several retrospective series demonstrating safety and feasibility of TRA for cerebrovascular procedures.[4–6] There is also higher patient satisfaction and preference with TRA in both coronary intervention and cerebrovascular angiograms,[5,14,15] likely due to earlier postprocedure ambulation, reduced length of stay, and less discomfort in the postprocedural recovery period with TRA when compared with TFA.

TRA provides a good option when the TFA may be difficult, especially in patients with severe obesity or severe atherosclerotic disease of the ilio-femoral arteries. For example, femoral or arch anatomy can make cerebral angiography prohibitively difficult in up to 5.1% of patients with acute ischemic stroke when TFA is used,

according to one series.[16] TRA can serve as an alternative approach in those patients. The RA can also serve as a second access site, when there is simultaneous need for multiple arterial access (eg, balloon test occlusion). Access to the left carotid artery in the bovine variant of arch (**Fig. 1**) and vertebral artery interventions might be more straightforward with TRA when compared with TFA. TRA is of utmost value in pregnant patients, where a catheter can be advanced via the RA to the cerebral vessels and bypassing the abdomen and pelvis, potentially limiting direct radiation exposure to the fetus.[17]

PATIENT SELECTION

The major limitation for TRA is the size of the RA. Hence, it is of importance to measure the RA diameter with ultrasound before the start of the procedure. When using an ultrasound for planning, be sure to have the patient in ideal conditions for a maximally dilated artery (eg, warm, calm) (see Technique section that follows). The ratio of RA diameter to outer diameter of sheath (A/S ratio) ideally should be >1 to avoid procedural limitations due to severe

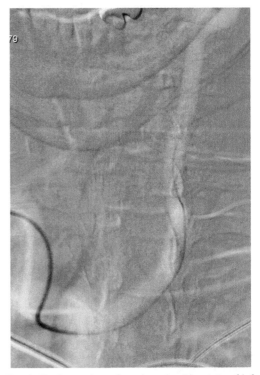

Fig. 1. Bovine variant of aortic arch with origin of left common carotid artery from innominate artery. Wire advancing in to left CCA without need of forming Simmons shape in arch.

spasm. Approximately 1.5 mm to 2.0 mm of cross-sectional diameter of RA is required for a 5-French sheath and diagnostic catheters. Cannulation and procedure can still be attempted with smaller RAs, but chances of vasospasm (Fig. 2) and TFA conversion are higher, especially in young women.[18,19] Embolization cases may require larger sheaths and intermediate catheters for support. For embolization cases in which the operator prefers to use large-bore sheaths (0.088 inner diameter [ID]), we would recommend that the arterial size is at least 2.3 mm in cross-sectional diameter.

Conventionally, the modified Allen test has been performed before radial access, to assess the collateral circulation to hand in the event of RA inadvertent occlusion. Barbeau and colleagues[20] developed a test using pulse oximetry to improve the sensitivity of the modified Allen test. Pulse oximetry is placed on the right thumb and the RA is compressed at the wrist for 2 minutes. Readings are categorized into 4 types (Fig. 3): A, no damping; B, slight damping of pulse tracing (most patients have this type); C, loss followed by recovery within 2 minutes; and D, no recovery of pulse tracing within 2 minutes.[20] A small minority of patients have type D pattern. These tests usually assess the integrity of superficial palmar arch, but despite incompleteness of this arch, hand ischemia is rare due to collaterals through the deep palmar arch. Recent large studies have shown poor predictive performance of this test for hand ischemia,[21] and routine preprocedural testing is no longer recommended.[22]

Anatomic variations of the aortic arch should be considered if the information is available from noninvasive vascular imaging. Right-sided TRA should be avoided in patients with aberrant origin of the right subclavian artery (Arteria Lusoria). Left-sided TRA can be used for those cases. On the other hand, access of left common carotid artery (CCA) is relatively easier with right TRA in bovine variants.

TECHNIQUE

Training of supporting staff, especially nurses and technicians, is pivotal in the preprocedural, intraprocedural, and postprocedural management of the patient with radial access. Patient reassurance, adequate sedation, proper table preparation, and optimal selection/preparation of dedicated equipment are indispensable. Right RA access is mostly used, with the exception of cases requiring specific access to the left vertebral artery or where aberrant origin of the right subclavian artery is noted. We routinely apply a combination of 5% topical lidocaine gel and 2% nitroglycerin ointment over the skin of the RA at the wrist, approximately 30 minutes before puncture. In addition, a warm pack or towel can be placed on the wrist and forearm to maximize dilation of the artery.

Room Setup

The patient is placed in supine position on the angiography table and the right arm is placed in supine position. Sometimes complete supine position of the forearm is not possible without increasing the distance away from the body significantly, particularly in older patients. In that case, partial supine position is acceptable or distal radial access can be pursued as described later in this article. The forearm and wrist should be elevated to the level of the groin to avoid a slope and catheters falling off the table (Fig. 4). Similarly, sufficient support with towels or other cushions may be placed on the extension board for catheter platform. Different

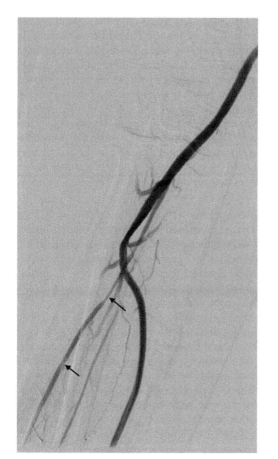

Fig. 2. Multifocal spasm in already small-caliber RA. Ulnar artery is larger in this patient.

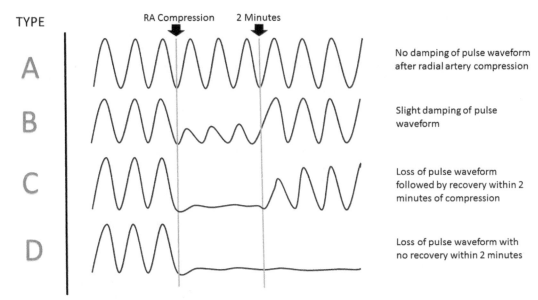

Fig. 3. Barbeau test. Pulse oximetry probe is placed on right thumb and RA is compressed at wrist for 2 minutes. Readings are categorized into 4 types: A, no damping; B, slight damping of pulse tracing (most patients have this type); C, loss followed by recovery within 2 minutes; and D, no recovery of pulse tracing within 2 minutes.

boards and extensions are commercially available to assist this position. Once positioned, sterile preparation of the right wrist is performed. The groins can also be prepared as a backup for failed radial access.

Cannulation

Before puncture, 2 to 3 mL of 1% lidocaine without epinephrine is infiltrated in the

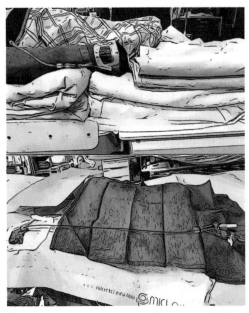

Fig. 4. Set up for transradial access. Notice the elevation of forearm and platform for catheters up to the level of body for flat surface.

subcutaneous tissue over the RA. The puncture site is usually just proximal to the styloid process of radius bone (Fig. 5). The mid or proximal forearm should be avoided to prevent compartment syndrome. Routine use of ultrasound is strongly recommended to avoid multiple attempts,[23] which increases the chances of vasospasm. Using a 20-gauge needle, the RA may be punctured with a single wall technique. If a counter puncture is used, the needle is slowly withdrawn back to the RA and a wire is advanced through needle (Video 1). A short 5-French sheath is typically used for diagnostic cerebral angiography.

Spasmolytics

Various combinations of spasmolytics, mainly calcium channel blockers, have been used.[18,24] A cocktail of spasmolytic medication can be slowly injected through the sheath (or through a microdilator), typically 2.5 mg verapamil and 200 µg of nitroglycerine or 3 to 5 mg of milrinone.[25] Hemodilution (aspirating a substantial amount of blood into the syringe) and slow injection should be performed, as these medications typically cause a burning sensation. Spasmolytics, especially nitroglycerine, can be repeated if there is persistent vasospasm as long as the blood pressure is in the desirable range. Some prefer to add heparin (3000–5000 units) in this cocktail to minimize RA occlusion, but this can significantly increase the burning sensation. Alternatively, it can be given via the intravenous route separately.

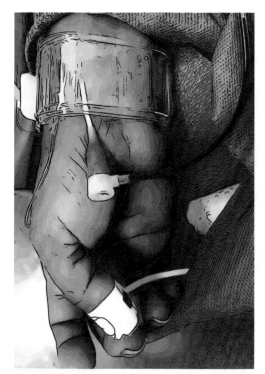

Fig. 5. Conventional radial artery puncture site. Transradial band for closure-sheath is partially withdrawn to snugly place band before inflation.

Catheterization

Although a 0.035 guide wire is typically used to transverse the RA, in cases of severe tortuosity, a 1.5-mm J-tip 0.035 hydrophilic coated guide wire (Terumo Interventional Systems, Somerset, NJ) or a 1.5-mm J-tip Rosen (nonhydrophilic) wire (Cook Medical, Bloomington, IN) may be used safely. A straight or angled tip hydrophilic guide wire should never be advanced without roadmap guidance. For diagnostic cerebral angiography, a Simmons-shaped catheter is most commonly used. We prefer a Simmons 2 catheter, which provides the ability to catheterize almost all major vessels for cerebral angiography. Alternatively, Simmons 1 or Simmons 3 can be used. The angio-table is rotated clockwise around 10° (−10) with single anteroposterior (AP) plane, to position the right forearm in the field of vision. The unformed Simmons catheter is advanced over guide wire to the proximal right subclavian artery under fluoroscopy. The angio-table is rotated back to neutral position and lateral plane is brought in for biplane angiography. The Simmons catheter needs to be formed to catheterize the vessels. There are different techniques to reform the Simmons shape; we favor to form in the descending aorta, which seems to be the safest of all because there would be minimized friction in the aortic arch.[5] The catheter is advanced to the descending aorta over the leading wire, until the proximal curve of the catheter is over the ascending aorta. The wire is then withdrawn into the catheter just before the proximal curve. Then, with a twisting motion, the catheter is pushed forward, which pushes the secondary curve into the ascending aorta and a Simmons shape is formed (Fig. 6, Video 2). The second most common way of reforming the shape is by tracking the catheter over the wire and deflecting on the aortic valve (Fig. 7, Video 3), which has a theoretic concern of distal embolism from the aortic valve. In a small percentage of cases, the wire can be

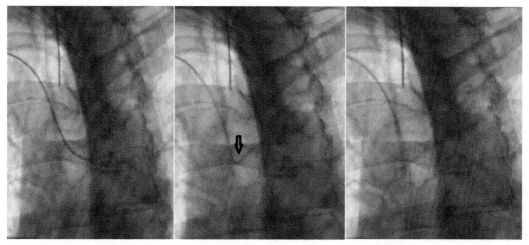

Fig. 6. Formation of Simmons shape in descending aorta. Advancing leading guide wire into descending aorta and then Simmons catheter over it, followed by withdrawing wire in subclavian artery and pushing catheter in ascending aorta (*arrow*) with twisting motion.

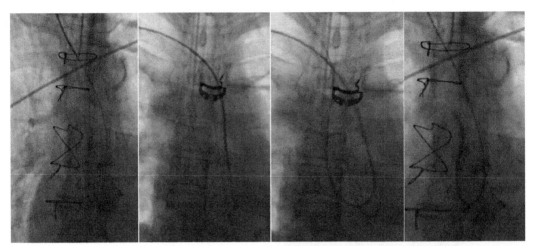

Fig. 7. Formation of Simmons shape in ascending aorta. With the catheter in subclavian artery, advance guidewire in ascending aorta, bounce off from aortic valve and advance catheter over the wire to reform the Simmons shape. Notice the significant purchase with wire before advancing catheter.

navigated directly into the right CCA or left CCA. In that case, the catheter can be advanced over the wire into the CCA without reforming the Simmons shape. Once the Simmons shape is formed, we generally catheterize the great vessels sequentially from left to right.

Sometimes it might be difficult to catheterize the left vertebral artery using a Simmons-2, in which case the catheter tip is kept as close to the vertebral artery origin as possible, the blood pressure cuff is inflated on the left arm, and contrast injection is performed in the left subclavian artery. Alternatively, Simmons 3 catheter, which has a longer distal end, can be used (Video 4). The catheter is pushed back in the arch to maintain its formed shape, and with the tip pointing upward, the catheter is advanced in the proximal left common carotid artery. Once a secondary curve is near the ostium of CCA, a road map is performed. The left internal carotid artery (ICA) and external carotid artery (ECA) are catheterized in a typical over-the-wire fashion, but it can be puffed from the internal to the external artery (Video 5). Caution should be exercised to have the CCA origin in an AP view, as sometimes an attempt to advance the catheter into the ICA over the wire can push the secondary curve back to arch, particularly in tortuous anatomy (Fig. 8). The Simmons catheter is slowly pulled and kept in its formed shape at the origin of the left carotid artery. It is then pushed and used to catheterize the right carotid system (Video 6). Of note, as mentioned previously, direct access of left CCA can be achieved, particularly in the bovine variant of arch, via right radial access, whereas it may be very challenging

via TFA (Video 7). The catheter is then withdrawn into the right subclavian artery, just distal to right CCA origin, and a road map is performed. The right vertebral artery is catheterized with the help of guide wire. For the right vertebral artery or right ICA/ECA, an angled Berenstein or vert catheter also can be used (Fig. 9, Video 8). A shapeable glidewire can be used to select the right (or even the left) common carotid arteries if an angled catheter is used and the angles are unfavorable.

Distal Radial Access

In recent years, distal radial access (dTRA) is getting more attention in an attempt to mitigate some of the limitations of conventional radial access.[6,26,27] By accessing the RA in the anatomic snuffbox, distal to the origin of superficial palmar branch, there is a theoretically lower risk of compromising the superficial palmar arch and less risk of hand ischemia. In addition, the forearm can be kept in mid-prone position right next to the body, which reduces discomfort because it is more ergonomic. In the event in which an operator has to use the left RA, it is very difficult to use the left conventional radial approach, as most of the neuro-angio suites are designed (controls and screen position), for the operator to be on the right side of the patient. In these cases, distal radial access is particularly useful to access the left vertebral artery procedures via the left forearm. The left forearm is kept partially flexed over the patient's abdomen with the hand close to the left groin, being then taped in place. The limiting factor for dTRA is the size of the artery, which can be

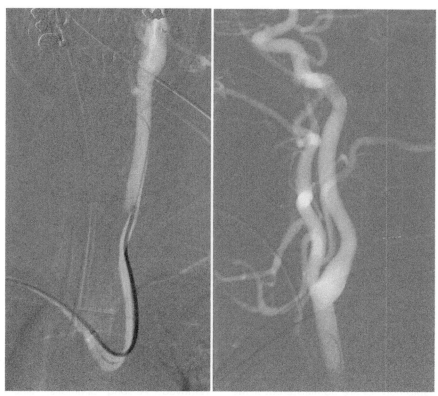

Fig. 8. Left CCA roadmap. AP view showing origin of artery with bend of catheter and lateral view showing bifurcation and majority of internal carotid artery.

up to 20% smaller in the snuffbox compared with the conventional radial puncture site. Smaller arterial size can predispose to severe spasm, which can result in higher conversion rates.[28]

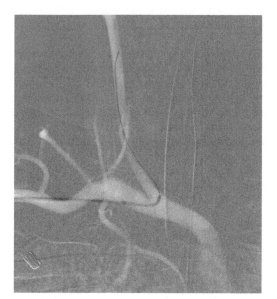

Fig. 9. Using angled tip catheter (Berenstein) to access right CCA. Same technique can be useful for right vertebral artery catheterization.

To perform dTRA, the hand is secured in a partly flexed and ulnar deviated position (**Fig. 10**). This brings the artery more superficial and straightens the arterial course. The rest of the technique is very similar to the conventional radial approach. For closure, there are dedicated compression bands available for dTRA, such as the PreludeSync distal radial band (Merit Medical, South Jordan, UT).

Interventions

TRA has been successfully used and described in a variety of cerebrovascular interventions, including mechanical thrombectomy (MT), aneurysm coiling, stent assisted coiling, flow diverter embolization, carotid artery stenting, and arteriovenous malformation embolization.[29–34] Historically but rarely, failure of TFA has conventionally led to potentially more dangerous access sites like carotid artery or brachial artery, especially during performing MT for acute ischemic stroke. TRA could be considered in those scenarios. By reducing anxiety and sympathetic drive, sedation and general anesthesia reduces the incidence of RA spasm,[35–37] which is convenient during intervention cases in which larger diameter sheaths are used. RA

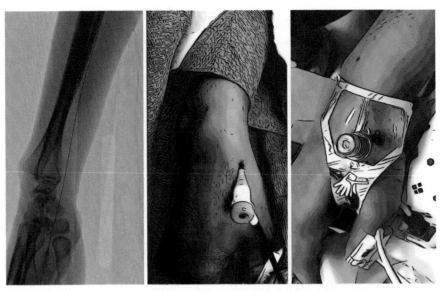

Fig. 10. Distal RA access in anatomic snuff box and closure with dedicated distal radial compression band.

cannulation is performed using a 6-French short sheath or 7-French thin-walled sheath. The sheath can be used to introduce a 0.070 ID system after spasmolytics are administered. If the RA size is between 2.0 mm and 2.3 mm, we prefer nontapered catheters like Envoy DA (Codman Neuro, Raynham, MA), for the ease of being able to use 0.058 intermediate catheter if needed. If the assistance of an intermediate catheter is not anticipated, then tapered catheters like Benchmark (Penumbra, Alameda, CA) also can be used. If the RA size is 2.3 mm or more, larger-bore catheters (examples mentioned later in this article) can be used. To do so, we recommend an exchange of the 6-French short sheath for large-bore catheters (ie, sheathless technique). We advise against use of large short sheaths like 8-French or higher for RA cannulation. After injecting spasmolytics through a short sheath, a 1.5-mm J-tipped wire is advanced up to the mid brachial artery and the short sheath is removed. A long sheath/guide catheter is then advanced in to the RA over the J wire (see Video 1). We prefer hydrophilic catheters like Infinity (Stryker Neurovascular, Fremont, CA); however, other catheters such as Neuron max (Penumbra), Fubuki (Asahi Intecc, Aichi, Japan), or Shuttle (Cook Medical, Bloomington, IN) can be used as long as the artery-to-sheath ratio is more than 1. Similar to TFA, a small skin incision might be necessary to advance the guide. Caution should be exercised by keeping the sharp end of the blade away from the artery and keeping the cut only

1 to 2 mm to prevent injury to the artery, which is very superficial. Once the guide catheter is advanced to the brachial artery, the J wire is removed. A long Simmons select catheter (130 cm; Penumbra) is advanced coaxially with 0.035 guidewire in the guide sheath and the Simmons shape is reformed in the arch as described previously, while keeping the guide sheath in the right subclavian artery. Once the Simmons catheter is in the common carotid artery, a guide wire is advanced into the intended artery (eg, left ICA). The long Simmons is advanced over the guide wire to the ICA and the guide catheter is then advanced over the Simmons catheter. Sometimes Simmons-select catheters do not easily advance over the wire and tend to herniate in the arch. In this scenario, while the guide wire is in the ICA and the select catheter is in the origin of the CCA, the guide sheath is advanced, first into the CCA before advancing the select catheter into the ICA (see Video 6). To access the right vertebral artery for posterior circulation interventions, an angled long vertebral or Berenstein catheter can be used.

Closure

Different external compression bands are available to close the radial arteriotomy site. They use an inflated air chamber against the puncture site for compression. The trans-radial band is snuggly fit over the puncture site and the air chamber is initially inflated with approximately 12 to 14 mL of air. The sheath is then completely removed. The air is slowly removed until visualization of bleeding, and 1 to 2 mL of air is briskly inserted back to stop the bleeding. This technique of patent hemostasis allows arterial flow while still maintaining hemostasis and minimizes the risk of RA occlusion.[38] Some data advocate compression of the ulnar artery for 1 to 2 minutes to force the blood through the RA and maintain its patency.[39] Different protocols are being used to deflate and remove the band. Our protocol is to remove 3 mL of air every 15 minutes, from the completion of the procedure as it coincides with the nursing protocol of postprocedural neuro-checks and vitals. If there is evidence of bleeding, air should be reinserted into the chamber to stop the bleeding. Overall, the longer external compression results, the higher chances of RA occlusion. With TRA, patients do not require bed rest (although the use of sedation should be considered), which results in significantly shorter recovery time compared with TFA.

LEARNING CURVE

Despite 2 decades of cardiology experience and well-demonstrated safety of TRA, the neurointervention world has been somewhat slow to embrace it as a first-line approach. There seems to be perceived difficulty of performing cerebral angiograms via TRA, mostly due to lack of training and awareness. There have been some data showing that experience with approximately 30 to 50 TRA cerebral angiograms is needed to become comfortable with TRA.[5,40] Over the learning curve, there is a reduction in crossover rate and fluoroscopy times, with better success with catheterizing all intended supra-aortic arteries.[5,40] No major complications have been reported in these 2 case series. The results are optimized with better patient selection, technicians' experience with position preparation/room setup, experience with RA cannulation and catheter navigation using Simmons shape catheter, and experience with managing RA spasm.

LIMITATIONS

Despite the advantages and feasibility, there are limitations of TRA. Some of them are cerebrovascular specific and some are related to the access site (Box 2). Early cardiology trials demonstrated that the risk of access failure and conversion were higher with the TRA (7.3% vs 2.0%).[41] However, more recent registries have shown a progressive reduction in the need for conversion (down to 1.5%), largely due to

---

Box 2
Limitations of TRA

- Vasospasm in patients with small radial artery
- Radial artery occlusion
- Limited ability to use larger systems like 9-French guide catheter
- Lack of radial specific cerebrovascular catheter systems

---

operator experience, improved techniques, and material.[9,42] RA spasm is noted from 4% to 20% of the cases.[35] RA occlusions have been reported to be from 0.8% to 33% in different series, but that can be reduced significantly with precautions described previously.[9,19,43–45] Apart from difficulty using the same RA for future access, clinical implications of RA occlusion are very limited.[46,47] Clinically relevant complications like hand ischemia requiring amputation and compartment syndrome are exceedingly rare.[19,48] Minor complications like extended access site pain, hematoma, or bruise are other possibilities.[49] There are few anatomic variations of the RA that operators should be aware of, such as high brachial artery bifurcation, radial or brachial artery loops, tortuosity of the RA, and the presence of an accessory RA. RA loops, which have an incidence of approximately 1%, can make it risky to advance the wire. In addition, if there is recurrent RA at the top of the loop, the wire can go into recurrent artery rather than RA, which may lead to perforation. For this reason, RA angiogram or roadmap is of paramount importance before advancing the wire. Arterial loops can be straightened by advancing a J wire or by advancing a micro-catheter over a micro-wire; however, in the case of persistent resistance it might be safer to change the access site. RA spasm is another well-known complication in up to 6% to 10% cases, as described previously. However, in many cases it can be relieved by spasmolytics and the procedure can be still completed. RA spasm that is refractory to conventional interventions (intra-arterial vasodilator therapy), sedation and analgesia, forearm warming, and reactive hyperemia may require general anesthesia or regional nerve block. For cerebrovascular angiography specifically, some challenging anatomies, such as the left vertebral artery, a right CCA with an acute angle, or a loop in the left CCA, may cause difficulty in catheterization of the vessels. This limitation is partly due to the current catheter systems that are designed to access supra-aortic vessels from the descending aorta. There is a lack of radial-specific catheters for cerebral angiography. Another physical limitation is not being able to use large catheter systems like 9-French balloon guide catheters for acute ischemic stroke. Furthermore, it is not well established that TRA is necessarily safer in patients with atherosclerotic disease involving the aortic arch for neuro-endovascular procedures. More data are needed to better understand the risks of TRA versus TFA in this population.

SUMMARY AND FUTURE DIRECTIONS

There is enough evidence to suggest that TRA is associated with a significantly lower incidence of bleeding, vascular complications, improved patient experience, and reduced health care costs. For these reasons TRA has become the standard approach in cardiac intervention. Interest in TRA has spiked in the neurointervention field. We are confident that with increasing experience, awareness, greater attention from industry, and advancement in technology, TRA will gain more popularity for cerebrovascular procedures.

SUPPLEMENTARY DATA

Supplementary data related to this article can be found online at https://doi.org/10.1016/j.iccl. 2019.08.008.

REFERENCES

1. Radner S. Thoracal aortography by catheterization from the radial artery; preliminary report of a new technique. Acta Radiol 1948;29(2):178–80.
2. Campeau L. Percutaneous radial artery approach for coronary angiography. Cathet Cardiovasc Diagn 1989;16(1):3–7.
3. Matsumoto Y, Hokama M, Nagashima H, et al. Transradial approach for selective cerebral angiography: technical note. Neurol Res 2000;22(6):605–8.
4. Park JH, Kim DY, Kim JW, et al. Efficacy of transradial cerebral angiography in the elderly. J Korean Neurosurg Soc 2013;53(4):213–7.
5. Snelling BM, Sur S, Shah SS, et al. Transradial cerebral angiography: techniques and outcomes. J Neurointerv Surg 2018;10(9):874–81.
6. Brunet MC, Chen SH, Sur S, et al. Distal transradial access in the anatomical snuffbox for diagnostic cerebral angiography. J Neurointerv Surg 2019;11(7): 710–3.
7. Jo KW, Park SM, Kim SD, et al. Is transradial cerebral angiography feasible and safe? A single center's experience. J Korean Neurosurg Soc 2010; 47(5):332–7.
8. Achenbach S, Ropers D, Kallert L, et al. Transradial versus transfemoral approach for coronary angiography and intervention in patients above 75 years of age. Catheter Cardiovasc Interv 2008;72(5): 629–35.
9. Jolly SS, Yusuf S, Cairns J, et al. Radial versus femoral access for coronary angiography and intervention in patients with acute coronary syndromes (RIVAL): a randomised, parallel group, multicentre trial. Lancet 2011;377(9775):1409–20.
10. Jolly SS, Amlani S, Hamon M, et al. Radial versus femoral access for coronary angiography or intervention and the impact on major bleeding and ischemic events: a systematic review and meta-analysis of randomized trials. Am Heart J 2009; 157(1):132–40.
11. Chase AJ, Fretz EB, Warburton WP, et al. Association of the arterial access site at angioplasty with transfusion and mortality: the M.O.R.T.A.L study (Mortality benefit Of Reduced Transfusion after percutaneous coronary intervention via the Arm or Leg). Heart 2008;94(8):1019–25.
12. Amoroso G, Sarti M, Bellucci R, et al. Clinical and procedural predictors of nurse workload during and after invasive coronary procedures: the potential benefit of a systematic radial access. Eur J Cardiovasc Nurs 2005;4(3):234–41.
13. Roussanov O, Wilson SJ, Henley K, et al. Cost-effectiveness of the radial versus femoral artery approach to diagnostic cardiac catheterization. J Invasive Cardiol 2007;19(8):349–53.
14. Satti SR, Vance AZ, Golwala SN, et al. Patient preference for transradial access over transfemoral access for cerebrovascular procedures. J Vasc Interv Neurol 2017;9(4):1–5.
15. Kok MM, Weernink MGM, von Birgelen C, et al. Patient preference for radial versus femoral vascular access for elective coronary procedures: the PRE-VAS study. Catheter Cardiovasc Interv 2018;91(1): 17–24.
16. Ribo M, Flores A, Rubiera M, et al. Difficult catheter access to the occluded vessel during endovascular treatment of acute ischemic stroke is associated with worse clinical outcome. J Neurointerv Surg 2013;5(Suppl 1):i70–3.
17. Shah SS, Snelling BM, Brunet MC, et al. Transradial mechanical thrombectomy for proximal middle cerebral artery occlusion in a first trimester pregnancy: case report and literature review. World Neurosurg 2018;120:415–9.
18. Chen CW, Lin CL, Lin TK, et al. A simple and effective regimen for prevention of radial artery spasm during coronary catheterization. Cardiology 2006; 105(1):43–7.
19. Uhlemann M, Möbius-Winkler S, Mende M, et al. The Leipzig prospective vascular ultrasound registry in radial artery catheterization: impact of sheath

size on vascular complications. JACC Cardiovasc Interv 2012;5(1):36–43.

20. Barbeau GR, Arsenault F, Dugas L, et al. Evaluation of the ulnopalmar arterial arches with pulse oximetry and plethysmography: comparison with the Allen's test in 1010 patients. Am Heart J 2004; 147(3):489–93.

21. van Leeuwen MAH, Hollander MR, van der Heijden DJ, et al. The ACRA anatomy study (assessment of disability after coronary procedures using radial access): a comprehensive anatomic and functional assessment of the vasculature of the hand and relation to outcome after transradial catheterization. Circ Cardiovasc Interv 2017;10(11) [pii:e005753].

22. Mason PJ, Shah B, Tamis-Holland JE, et al. An update on radial artery access and best practices for transradial coronary angiography and intervention in acute coronary syndrome: a scientific statement from the American Heart Association. Circ Cardiovasc Interv 2018;11(9):e000035.

23. Seto AH, Roberts JS, Abu-Fadel MS, et al. Real-time ultrasound guidance facilitates transradial access: RAUST (Radial Artery access with Ultrasound Trial). JACC Cardiovasc Interv 2015;8(2):283–91.

24. Varenne O, Jégou A, Cohen R, et al. Prevention of arterial spasm during percutaneous coronary interventions through radial artery: the SPASM study. Catheter Cardiovasc Interv 2006;68(2):231–5.

25. Levy EI, Boulos AS, Fessler RD, et al. Transradial cerebral angiography: an alternative route. Neurosurgery 2002;51(2):335–40 [discussion: 340–2].

26. Kiemeneij F. Left distal transradial access in the anatomical snuffbox for coronary angiography (ldTRA) and interventions (ldTRI). EuroIntervention 2017;13(7):851–7.

27. Patel P, Majmundar N, Bach I, et al. Distal Transradial Access in the Anatomic Snuffbox for Diagnostic Cerebral Angiography. AJNR Am J Neuroradiol 2019;40(9):1526–8.

28. Koutouzis M, Kontopodis E, Tassopoulos A, et al. Distal versus traditional radial approach for coronary angiography. Cardiovasc Revasc Med 2018; 20(8):678–80.

29. Ruzsa Z, Nemes B, Pintér L, et al. A randomised comparison of transradial and transfemoral approach for carotid artery stenting: RADCAR (RADial access for CARotid artery stenting) study. EuroIntervention 2014;10(3):381–91.

30. Daou B, Chalouhi N, Tjoumakaris S, et al. Alternative access for endovascular treatment of cerebrovascular diseases. Clin Neurol Neurosurg 2016; 145:89–95.

31. Haussen DC, Nogueira RG, DeSousa KG, et al. Transradial access in acute ischemic stroke intervention. J Neurointerv Surg 2016;8(3):247–50.

32. Sur S, Snelling B, Khandelwal P, et al. Transradial approach for mechanical thrombectomy in anterior circulation large-vessel occlusion. Neurosurg Focus 2017;42(4):E13.

33. Chen SH, Snelling BM, Shah SS, et al. Transradial approach for flow diversion treatment of cerebral aneurysms: a multicenter study. J Neurointerv Surg 2019;11(8):796–800.

34. Nardai S, Végh E, Óriás V, et al. Feasibility of distal radial access for carotid interventions: the RADCAR-DISTAL pilot study. EuroIntervention 2019. [Epub ahead of print].

35. Ho HH, Jafary FH, Ong PJ. Radial artery spasm during transradial cardiac catheterization and percutaneous coronary intervention: incidence, predisposing factors, prevention, and management. Cardiovasc Revasc Med 2012;13(3):193–5.

36. Pullakhandam NS, Yang ZJ, Thomas S, et al. Unusual complication of transradial catheterization. Anesth Analg 2006;103(3):794–5.

37. Deftereos S, Giannopoulos G, Raisakis K, et al. Moderate procedural sedation and opioid analgesia during transradial coronary interventions to prevent spasm: a prospective randomized study. JACC Cardiovasc Interv 2013;6(3):267–73.

38. Pancholy S, Coppola J, Patel T, et al. Prevention of radial artery occlusion-patent hemostasis evaluation trial (PROPHET study): a randomized comparison of traditional versus patency documented hemostasis after transradial catheterization. Catheter Cardiovasc Interv 2008;72(3):335–40.

39. Koutouzis MJ, Maniotis CD, Avdikos G, et al. ULnar artery transient compression facilitating radial artery patent hemostasis (ULTRA): a novel technique to reduce radial artery occlusion after transradial coronary catheterization. J Invasive Cardiol 2016; 28(11):451–4.

40. Zussman BM, Tonetti DA, Stone J, et al. Maturing institutional experience with the transradial approach for diagnostic cerebral arteriography: overcoming the learning curve. J Neurointerv Surg 2019. [Epub ahead of print].

41. Agostoni P, Biondi-Zoccai GG, de Benedictis ML, et al. Radial versus femoral approach for percutaneous coronary diagnostic and interventional procedures; systematic overview and meta-analysis of randomized trials. J Am Coll Cardiol 2004;44(2):349–56.

42. Singh S, Singh M, Grewal N, et al. Transradial vs transfemoral percutaneous coronary intervention in ST-segment elevation myocardial infarction: a systemic review and meta-analysis. Can J Cardiol 2016;32(6):777–90.

43. Kiemeneij F, Laarman GJ, Odekerken D, et al. A randomized comparison of percutaneous transluminal coronary angioplasty by the radial, brachial

and femoral approaches: the access study. J Am Coll Cardiol 1997;29(6):1269–75.

44. Stella PR, Kiemeneij F, Laarman GJ, et al. Incidence and outcome of radial artery occlusion following transradial artery coronary angioplasty. Cathet Cardiovasc Diagn 1997;40(2):156–8.

45. Hildick-Smith DJ, Lowe MD, Walsh JT, et al. Coronary angiography from the radial artery–experience, complications and limitations. Int J Cardiol 1998;64(3):231–9.

46. Sciahbasi A, Rigattieri S, Sarandrea A, et al. Radial artery occlusion and hand strength after percutaneous coronary procedures: results of the HANGAR study. Catheter Cardiovasc Interv 2016;87(5):868–74.

47. van der Heijden DJ, van Leeuwen MAH, Ritt MJPF, et al. Hand sensibility after transradial arterial access: an observational study in patients with and without radial artery occlusion. J Vasc Interv Radiol 2019. [Epub ahead of print].

48. Tizon-Marcos H, Barbeau GR. Incidence of compartment syndrome of the arm in a large series of transradial approach for coronary procedures. J Interv Cardiol 2008;21(5):380–4.

49. Jaroenngarmsamer T, Bhatia KD, Kortman H, et al. Procedural success with radial access for carotid artery stenting: systematic review and meta-analysis. J Neurointerv Surg 2019. [Epub ahead of print].

Vascular Complications of the Wrist
Prevention and Management

Samir B. Pancholy, MD[a],*, Gaurav A. Patel, MD[a],
Sanjay C. Shah, MD[b], Tejas M. Patel, MD[b]

KEYWORDS

- Transradial access • Access site-related complications • Prevention and treatment

---

KEY POINTS

- Transradial access has increased in utilization and has been shown to be superior compared with transfemoral access.
- Although infrequent, several transradial access site-related complications occur.
- By understanding potential mechanisms related to these complications, several prevention and treatment strategies can be implemented to mitigate adverse outcomes.

INTRODUCTION

Compared with transfemoral access, transradial access (TRA) has been shown to significantly reduce the incidence of access site–related complications, improved patient comfort, lower procedural cost, and in certain subsets, improve hard outcomes.[1] Although complications are infrequent, several complications specific to TRA occur. In this document, the authors describe the prevalence, the likely mechanism of causation of these complications, strategies for prevention, and treatment of these complications.

RADIAL ARTERY SPASM

The most common functional complication of TRA is radial artery spasm. High density of alpha receptor in the muscular radial artery wall,[2] as well as tactile stimulation due to hardware transit in the setting of a hyperadrenergic state caused by an anxious patient with inadequate sedation, usually leads to spasm of the radial artery.

Puncture-Related Spasm

In view of the small caliber of radial artery as well as a significantly higher wall thickness-to-lumen diameter ratio, accessing the radial artery is somewhat challenging, and a learning curve has been observed.[3] Because the radial artery lumen is significantly smaller than the other arterial access locations, successful advancement of guide wire frequently is difficult. Failed cannulation after needle puncture may lead to loss of radial pulse. Severe spasm of the distal radial artery because of multiple failed punctures is usually observed during the operator's initial learning curve. Because of a small-diameter lumen, after puncturing the anterior wall and entering the lumen, stabilization of the cannula is difficult, and frequently due to the antegrade flow of blood, the cannula is pushed back out of the lumen. Hence, wire advancement is either not possible or could be subintimal. Instrumentation-related tactile stimulation of the radial artery wall, being rich in alpha receptor density, has a low threshold for developing spasm. Spasm leads to a resultant loss

---

Disclosure Statement: The authors have no relevant disclosures to reveal.
[a] Division of Cardiology, The Wright Center for Graduate Medical Education, 111 North Washington Avenue, Scranton, PA 18503, USA; [b] Division of Cardiology, Apex Heart Institute, G-K Mondeal Business Park, Near Gurudwara Govindham Thaltej, Sarkhej–Gandhinagar Highway, Ahmedabad, Gujarat 380054, India
* Corresponding author. 401 North State Street, Clarks Summit, PA 18411.
E-mail address: pancholy8@gmail.com

Intervent Cardiol Clin 9 (2020) 87–97
https://doi.org/10.1016/j.iccl.2019.08.002

of pulsatile sensation, making further attempts more difficult.

Prevention

The best strategy to prevent failed puncture-related spasm is to aim for first-pass successful access. As the 2-point discrimination of the human fingertip is roughly in the same vicinity as the diameter of the radial artery, early in the learning process first-pass first-attempt puncture could be difficult. Use of ultrasonography is recommended to maximize first-attempt success in cannulation.[4] Counterpuncture technique, by the way of transfixation of the radial artery, has also been shown to improve first-attempt successful cannulation.[5]

Treatment

If the radial artery in the distal forearm has developed spasm and the pulsation is either very faint or nonpalpable, several strategies could be used to relieve the spasm. Time is one of the best solutions if available, although waiting for the pulsatile sensation to normalize could frequently take long durations of time. Administration of vasodilators systemically, such as sublingual nitroglycerin administration or intravenous nitroglycerin administration, is successful in relieving failed puncture-related spasm, although by default, will cause systemic effects of these vasodilator treatments. Local subcutaneous injection of 200 μg nitroglycerin in the vicinity of the failed attempted puncture has also been shown to provide rapid resolution of radial artery spasm and has not been associated with systemic side effects.[6]

Radial Artery Spasm After Obtaining Transradial Access

Spasm may occur after obtaining successful TRA, beyond the introducer sheath. In most cases, some spasm occurs, although it is not perceived by the operator or the patient, and the procedure is not interrupted as a result of minor spasm. Significant spasm is noted in younger patients, more in women compared with men, and in patients who do not receive sedation. Nonhydrophilic introducer sheaths as well as multiple catheter exchanges increase the incidence of spasm.[7] Because of the lack of consensus of definition of radial artery spasm, the incidence of radial artery spasm in the literature varies from 0.3% to 14%. Spasm leading to inability to advance hardware across the radial artery occurs in 0.7% of patients.[8] In general, treatment with additional intraarterial vasodilators is successful in relieving spasm. Focal spasm is more forgiving

from the standpoint of resolution after treatment as well as from its ability to obstruct transit. Long segments of spasm usually require dedicated treatment and lead to prolongation of procedure duration.

Prevention

By tackling each of the mechanistic influences, the best strategy for prevention of radial artery spasm should include the following:

A. A calm and quiet catheterization laboratory environment with a confident team, including the operator as well as the ancillary professionals.
B. Administration of anxiolytics and sedation to the patient before the procedure.
C. Use of hydrophilic introducer sheath, which has been shown to lower the incidence of radial artery spasm. Sheath length has not been found to be associated with the incidence of radial artery spasm.
D. Limiting the number of catheter exchanges might reduce the incidence of radial artery spasm.

Treatment

Once radial artery spasm has occurred, the best strategies to relieve spasm include the following:

A. Administration of intraarterial vasodilators, either nitrates (nitroglycerin or nitroprusside) or calcium channel blockers (verapamil, diltiazem, or nicardipine), if hemodynamics allow (Fig. 1).
B. Administration of additional sedation if the patient is anxious.
C. Warming up the room temperature as well as application of local warm compresses to the forearm.
D. An adverse anatomic substrate should be suspected if spasm is not improving despite above interventions, because frequently these instances of "refractory spasm" are not spasm but aberrant anatomy leading to impediment in hardware transit through the radial artery.

PERFORATION AND HEMATOMAS

Radial artery perforation occurs because of several mechanisms. The most common mechanism of a small perforation is inadvertent advancement of the tip of a guide wire into a small muscular branch while traversing the radial artery in the forearm. Entry of this metallic or hydrophilic guide wire into a small muscular side branch leads to fenestration of this small branch

BEFORE

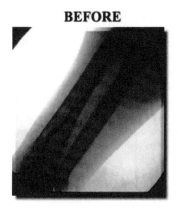

AFTER

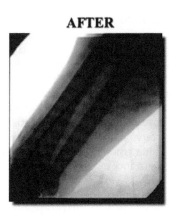

Fig. 1. Treatment of radial artery spasm with vasodilators. Radial artery spasm was noted after obtaining TRA (*before*). Verapamil was administered intraarterially with successful resolution of spasm (*after*).

that then leads to extravasation. In most instances, the patient reports a fleeting episode of localized pain that subsequently quickly resolves and frequently goes unattended. High index of suspicion with attention to any discomfort in the forearm no matter how trivial and transient it may be may lead to immediate detection and subsequent treatment of this complication with excellent outcomes.

The other mechanism of perforation is forceful advancement of hardware through abnormal lumen as a result of either spasm or aberrant anatomy. Because of large transitions, the "razor effect" is frequently operational and leads to deep medial dissections and subsequent perforation if undue force is used (Fig. 2). Perforations if not attended promptly lead to extravasation and accumulation in the interosseous compartment, which being a closed space could lead to rapid increase in compartmental pressure

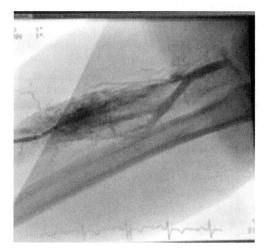

Fig. 2. Radial artery perforation. Forceful advancement of hardware through abnormal lumen resulted in radial artery perforation leading to extravasation and accumulation in the interosseous compartment.

leading to injury to the nerves as well as other components of the compartment, with catastrophic long-term consequences if uncorrected.

Prevention

The most important routine to follow while traversing the forearm arterial vasculature is to have a very low threshold to perform a low-pressure radial artery angiogram if any resistance is encountered or if the patient reports any pain in the forearm. Use of specialized equipment, such as hydrophilic angled-tip guide wires and more steerable guide wires, is specifically discouraged in the absence of preceding angiography to define the arterial terrain. Alternatively, a 1.5-mm radius J-tip 0.035-inch hydrophilic wire may be used without prior angiography. If difficult anatomy is encountered, using techniques that decrease wire to catheter transition, such as telescoping catheter use, or balloon-assisted tracking,[9] leads to a near total elimination of the razor effect and hence atraumatic transit of hardware through a hostile segment without causing vessel trauma.

Treatment

A. If low-pressure radial angiography is performed, perforation will be detected before arterial access is abandoned. In most instances, the best modality of treatment of radial artery perforation is to maintain guide wire access, advance a catheter proximal to the perforated segment, and allow enough dwell time for the artery to tamponade itself from the inside. This leads to adequate closure of the perforation rent leading to cessation of extravasation in most cases. Reversal of anticoagulation is usually not necessary, and in most instances, a diagnostic or interventional procedure could proceed without interruption as long as the catheter remains across the perforated segment. In the authors' experience, a dwell time of 20 to 30 minutes has proven to be adequate in sealing the perforations successfully. Larger perforations that do not seal after prolonged intraarterial catheter dwell time might be caused by long lacerations of radial artery wall and may need dedicated repair either using a covered stent, or in rare instances, operative repair.

B. Perforations recognized after removal of introducer sheath from the radial artery pose a more difficult problem in view of the lack of clarity of the mechanism and location of vessel wall injury. In this instance, the only option of treatment is extrinsic compression of the potential perforation site with the aim to prevent extravasation and hence increase in pressure in the interosseous space (Fig. 3). High index of suspicion is needed to immediately treat this possibility. *Any pain in the forearm reported by the patient after the procedure should be taken very seriously*, and a presumed perforation should be treated with extrinsic compression of the radial artery especially if the forearm appears to be swollen. A preprocedural evaluation of the forearm morphology is very helpful in aiding the operator in detection of postprocedural hematomas. Any significant delay in immediate recognition and treatment of this perforation-related hematoma formation could lead to a catastrophic complication of compartment syndrome frequently leading to irreversible damage to the forearm

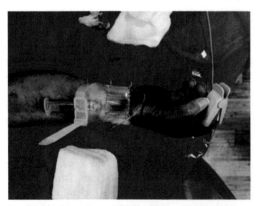

Fig. 3. Applying focused pressure to prevent expansion of hematoma. Extrinsic focused compression of the potential perforation site was applied with the aim to prevent extravasation and accumulation in the interosseous compartment.

nerves with loss of function of the hand if not treated promptly. In the event of occurrence of forearm hematoma, neurologic function as well as perfusion of the digits should be very closely monitored. This is 1 complication of TRA whereby vascular surgery consultation should be obtained on an emergent basis. Any decrease in neurologic function of the digits should lead to immediate operative compression of a forearm hematoma using either fasciotomy or other means.

Perforations Proximal to Radial Artery

Brachial artery perforation is certainly possible, although most brachial artery perforations are avulsed, accessory, or high-insertion radial arteries owing to the forceful catheter advancement. Once again, these could be prevented by attending to any tactile feeling of resistance to advancement of hardware. In the event of avulsion of a high-takeoff radial artery, depending on the location of avulsion and the diameter of the high-takeoff radial artery, operative repair may be needed. Because the brachial artery is an end artery, compression with the intent to stop flow is not an option.

Perforations in the subclavian and innominate artery sectors are caused by hydrophilic guide wire–related perforations of smaller branches due to inadvertent forceful entry and need to be treated with covered stent placement, because these sites are frequently noncompressible.

Hand Hematoma

This complication is a unique entity that has surfaced with the use of dorsal radial artery access for endovascular procedures.[10] It is likely caused by similar mechanisms as the perforations in other arteries described above. The treatment is extrinsic compression with resolution of the mass effect caused by the hematoma as well as cessation of extravasation. Long-term consequences of this complication are largely unknown.

For the purposes of communication with other providers and record-keeping, the EASY hematoma grading system may be used.[11]

HARDWARE ENTRAPMENT

Although very infrequent, one of the most unnerving instances in the catheterization laboratory is the inability to remove catheters and introducers from the access artery at the end of the procedure. This is largely caused by spasm, although once again, focal spasm does not cause impediment of hardware transit when entering as well as upon withdrawal. Long areas of spasm are usually present when entrapment occurs. In addition to spasm, in most instances, abnormal anatomic substrate is present. Entrapment should be suspected when upon attempted withdrawal of the catheter or introducer the patient experiences pain, and a linear indentation is observed on the skin overlying the path taken by a superficial artery (Fig. 4).

Prevention

Minimization of tactile stimulation of the arterial wall by limiting the number of catheter exchanges and paying careful attention to the catheter-to-artery ratio lowers the incidence of catheter entrapment. Using hydrophilic equipment, especially introducers, is also essential in preventing entrapment. Careful attention to tactile feel while advancing the guide wire, in order to detect abnormal anatomy upfront, eliminates inadvertent placement of hardware through aberrant anatomy and hence eliminates the subsequent problem of entrapment. Other measures to minimize the tendency of spasm, such as adequate sedation as well as a calm environment in the catheterization laboratory and routine use of intraarterial vasodilator "cocktail," may further lower the probability of entrapment. Shorter procedure durations may further decrease the likelihood of entrapment.

Treatment

In view of the fact that radial artery spasm is the likely culprit mechanism, all measures known to reduce radial spasm are effective in relieving entrapment. These include the following:

A. Administration of intraarterial and, if necessary, systemic vasodilators, such as nitroglycerin, calcium channel blockers, as well as other vasodilators. Maximization of sedation as well as the application of warm compresses to the forearm and increasing the temperature of the catheterization suite may help.

B. Exploitation of local physiology to cause profound local vasodilatation is an attractive option, if these initial simple treatments are not effective. A technique described earlier,[12] using the principle of ischemia and flow-mediated vasodilatation, has been shown to be effective in relieving entrapment with high success rates. In this technique, a sphygmomanometer cuff is applied to the proximal upper arm with the intent to occlude flow in the axillary or brachial artery, by inflating the cuff to pressures exceeding the systolic blood pressure. The cuff is left inflated at this pressure for approximately 5 minutes, leading to mild ischemia of the distal extremity. It is usually well tolerated for this duration. Upon relieving the pressure from the cuff and reestablishing antegrade flow in the arterial circuit, a profound wave of vasodilatation in the distal arterial circulation is observed with frequent release of the entrapped hardware (Fig. 5). This technique has several benefits, including its high success rate as well as lack of systemic adverse effects.

C. In the event of failure of abovementioned maneuvers in relieving entrapment,

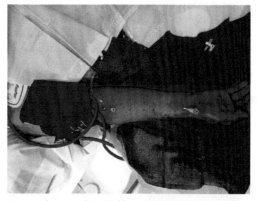

Fig. 5. Flow-mediated dilatation technique to relieve entrapment. A sphygmomanometer cuff is applied to the proximal upper arm, and the cuff is inflated to suprasystemic pressure. Upon relieving the pressure from the cuff, antegrade flow is established with a profound wave of vasodilatation in the distal arterial circulation resulting in release of the entrapped hardware.

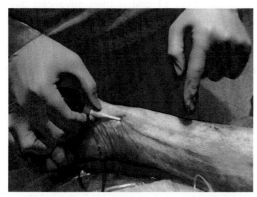

Fig. 4. Entrapped sheath with attempted removal. Entrapment is suspected when upon attempted withdrawal of the catheter or introducer, a linear indentation is observed on the skin overlying the path taken by a superficial artery.

administration of deep sedation using propofol in the setting of monitored anesthesia care or administration of general anesthesia may be necessary to relieve entrapment. Although local nerve blocks, such as brachial plexus block, have been described in isolated instances to be effective, in an anticoagulated patient, these are usually not advisable.

It is very important to not apply excessive force to remove the entrapped hardware. Application of excessive force could lead to a serious complication of total avulsion of the arterial wall, which has very serious consequences.[13]

CATHETER KINKING

In patients with significant tortuosity of the of upper extremity and central vasculature, catheter manipulation, especially rotational torque application, is difficult, and hence, operators may frequently apply torsion that may not be transmitted to the proximal catheter, resulting in kinking of the catheter. Kinking not only results in interruption of the continuity of the lumen of the catheter making the catheter lose its utility as a conduit for transit of contrast or other hardware, but in many instances, it folds upon itself, developing a larger profile that leads to inability to advance or remove the catheter from the artery (Fig. 6A). Forceful movement of a kinked catheter could lead to severe luminal and deeper injury to the artery and should be avoided.

Prevention
While navigating with a catheter through tortuous anatomy, caution should be advised when applying rotational torque with careful attention paid to the amount of torque applied in 1 direction and systematic offsetting by rotating the catheter in the opposite direction. Frequently, leaving a guide wire in the catheter

lumen while applying torque maybe necessary to increase the efficacy of torque transmission as well as prevent the catheter from kinking. Finally, the operator should carefully observe pressure tracings, because dampening of pressure is often an early sign of catheter kinking.

Treatment
A. If the catheter proximal to the kink segment is in a superficial location (eg, upper arm or forearm), external compression of the proximal segment of the catheter, using either manual pressure or application of a sphygmomanometer cuff inflated to suprasystemic pressures, may lead to immobilization of the proximal segment of the catheter, after which if opposite torque is applied the kink could be "undone," and the catheter successfully removed without further arterial trauma.

B. Similar immobilization of the proximal shaft of the catheter could be achieved by using a snare advanced to the proximal portion of the catheter from an alternative access site. Once the proximal portion of the catheter is anchored by the snare and immobilized, opposite torque is applied once again to "undo" the kink after which the proximal portion of the catheter is released from the snare and the catheter is successfully removed from the artery.

C. An elegant "swallowing-the-kink" technique may be used to remove kinked catheters. A larger catheter or introducer that is larger than the kinked catheter in size (eg, 6F introducer for 5F kinked catheter) is placed over the kinked catheter after cutting off the catheter hub. The introducer (preferably longer than 11 cm) is then advanced over the distal shaft of the kinked catheter, and under fluoroscopic guidance, the kinked segment is carefully traversed by advancing

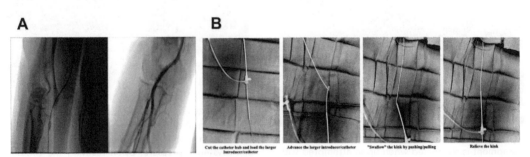

Fig. 6. (A) Catheter kinking. Kinking of the catheter due to inadvertent advancement. (B) Relieving catheter kink by "swallowing technique." Using a larger catheter/introducer to relieve the kinked catheter by telescoping the larger diameter catheter over the kinked catheter. ([A] Courtesy Rajiv Gulati, MD, Mayo Clinic, Rochester, MN.)

the larger introducer over the kinked segment of the catheter. Once the kink is relieved, the guide wire is advanced once back bleeding is observed, and the hardware is removed (Fig. 6B). When advancing a guide wire through a kinked catheter once the kink is relieved, careful attention to the presence of back bleeding before advancing the guide wire will prevent potential embolization of thrombus that may have formed in the kinked catheter because of stasis.

RADIAL ARTERY PSEUDOANEURYSM

Pseudoaneurysms (PA) occur in 0.03% of patients undergoing TRA.[14] They are mostly observed in patients with diseased radial artery, such as very elderly patients with high atherosclerotic burden, patients with chronic kidney disease, or in the setting of continued long-term systemic anticoagulant therapy. They usually occur a few days after the procedure with the usual presentation of a tender pulsatile swelling at the puncture site with a palpable thrill or audible bruit (Fig. 7). Ecchymoses to a varying degree are noted surrounding the PA. In view of the risk of dehiscence and subsequent massive bleeding, despite their apparent tolerance, they need to be treated with the intent to definitively eliminate flow in the PA sac and seal the rent in the radial artery.

Prevention

Careful attention to hemostasis, with adequate duration of compression allowing for stabilization of the occlusive thrombus plug, is essential in decreasing the probability of subsequent PA

formation. Because many of the operating mechanisms in development of PA after TRA are patient substrate–related, such as need for systemic anticoagulant therapy and so on, preventive measures are limited.

A localized swelling at the puncture site should be carefully examined with palpation for a thrill and auscultation to assess for presence of a bruit with a very low threshold to perform ultrasonography to evaluate the swelling. Documentation of flow in the PA sac with a rent in the radial artery wall is essential for the diagnosis of PA. Definitive treatment is needed once the diagnosis is made.

Treatment

A. Application of extrinsic pressure, using hemostatic compression devices, such as balloon inflatable and other bands, with the intent to interrupt flow across the rent in the radial artery and in that PA sac is frequently effective in thrombosing the PA.

B. Larger PA not responding to compression manually or by using a band, with or without ultrasound guidance, may need ultrasound-guided thrombin injection. Because of its superficial location, visualization of the neck as well as the contents of the PA is very easily accomplished using duplex ultrasound (Fig. 8). Using a micropuncture needle, the PA sack is entered, and the needle tip is directed away from the neck of the aneurysm (Fig. 9). After a test injection of sailing under ultrasound guidance, 50 µg thrombin is injected as a 1-mL solution in the aneurysm sac, while compressing the neck of the aneurysm. Within 5 to 10 minutes, the echogenicity of the contents of the PA sack are noted to increase, with

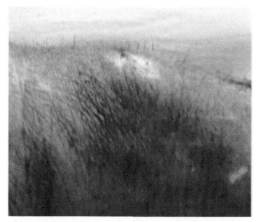

Fig. 7. Radial artery PA. Tender pulsatile swelling at the puncture site with a palpable thrill and audible bruit indicating formation of radial artery PA.

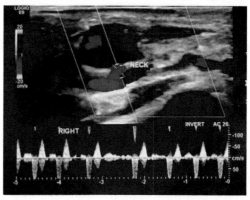

Fig. 8. Ultrasound of radial artery PA. Visualization of the neck and contents of the radial artery PA using duplex ultrasound.

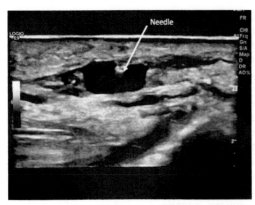

Fig. 9. Entry into PA with a micropuncture needle. Using a micropuncture needle, the PA sack is entered, and the needle tip is directed away from the neck of the aneurysm.

the ultrasound signature of the PA sack changing from a deep black appearance to a gray appearance (Fig. 10). This is a morphologic marker of thrombosis of the PA sack. At this point, with gradual release in pressure on the neck of the PA, complete lack of flow is frequently observed. Thrombin should not be injected without compression of the neck and cessation of flow to prevent distal ischemic complications due to thrombin.

C. PA with a wide neck may pose a particular challenge with failure of abovementioned treatments. Surgical excision of the PA with subsequent repair of the rent in the radial artery is highly effective and usually could be performed under local anesthesia.

D. In those circumstances whereby surgical option is not available, percutaneous extirpation is possible.[15] Flow across the

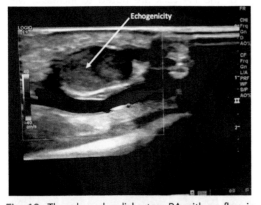

Fig. 10. Thrombosed radial artery PA with no flow in the sac. Thrombosis of the PA sac is noted within 5 to 10 minutes of thrombin injection with change in echogenicity of the content of the PA sac from deep black to gray appearance.

neck of the PA could be interrupted by placement of an introducer sheath in the radial artery from a location distal to the original puncture site, traversing the segment with the PA with the introducer sheath interrupting flow across the neck of the PA. The introducer sheath is then left in place for 6 to 8 hours with a traditional arterial line pressure flush apparatus commonly used in the intensive care setting attached to the introducer sheath to prevent sheath thrombosis. After 6 to 8 hours, the introducer sheath is withdrawn distal to the PA sac, and a low-pressure angiogram is performed to assess the status of the PA. Thrombosis of the PA sack with sealing of the rent of the radial artery may be observed.

RADIAL ARTERY OCCLUSION

Radial artery occlusion (RAO) is the most common structural complication of TRA. It occurs in 2% to 10% of patients undergoing TRA. RAO is likely caused by intimal injury caused by the hardware at the puncture site and beyond, in conjunction with stasis created by placement of the hardware as well as subsequent hemostatic compression leading to thrombus formation and subsequent rapid organization with obliteration of the lumen. Because of extensive macrocollateralization as well as microcollateralization in the forearm, acute ischemia due to the RAO is usually not observed. The isolated reports of digital ischemia published in the literature are presumed to be due to embolic in cause. Despite its lack of potential to cause ischemic complications, it is of paramount importance to prevent RAO in order to preserve the radial artery for future access as well as prevention of other unmeasurable consequences of RAO.

Prevention

Several strategies have been found to be effective in lowering the incidence of RAO, including the following:

A. In an effort to reduce intimal trauma, the lowest profile hardware necessary to achieve the goal of the endovascular procedure should be used. The caliber of the hardware should be preferably smaller than the lumen diameter of the radial artery.

B. Use of intraprocedural parenteral anticoagulation administered at adequate doses is essential in preventing RAO. Several datasets have demonstrated excellent efficacy of unfractionated heparin

(UFH), with a dose-response relationship with higher efficacy noted with higher doses.[16,17] Other anticoagulants, such as enoxaparin and bivalirudin,[18] have also been shown to be effective. The currently recommended dose based on available evidence is 5000 units or 50 units/kg of UFH in patients at the extremes of weight, administered as a bolus, either intraarterially or intravenously during the procedure.

C. The most effective strategy for prevention of RAO is careful attention to avoid interruption of radial artery flow during hemostatic compression of the radial artery.[19] This method, termed "patent hemostasis," has been proposed as a "best practice" and is highly effective in significantly lowering the incidence of RAO without any adverse effects.[20] Hemostatic compression is initiated by any methodology preferred by the operator, and after establishment of initial hemostasis, the hemostatic compression pressure is titrated to the least necessary pressure applied to achieve dry hemostasis. If using a compression device, the device is left in place at this level of compression pressure, with frequent observation of the puncture site as well as the distal digits for adequacy of hemostasis as well as presence of antegrade radial artery flow, respectively.

D. Longer duration of compression is associated with a higher rate of RAO, and hence, excessively long compression durations should be avoided.[21,22] Very short duration of compression may be associated with rebound bleeding. Rebound bleeding is the strongest predictor of RAO as demonstrated in the recent randomized trial[23] and should be avoided.

E. The arterial circulation in the forearm comprises 2 large arterial conduits, the radial and the ulnar artery, with macroscopic as well as microcommunications between these 2 arteries. In view of these communications and hence interdependence, flow dynamics in one of these vessels affects the flow dynamics in the other vessel. This anatomic and physiologic substrate could be exploited to maximize the probability of radial artery patency while performing radial hemostatic compression. Compression of the ipsilateral ulnar artery has been shown to increase the radial artery velocity time integral by nearly 40%.[24] Because flow increase is associated with a lower probability of thrombosis, this increase in radial artery flow could be recruited to further prevent RAO. Recent observational[25] and randomized studies[26] have demonstrated the efficacy of concomitant ipsilateral ulnar artery compression in further lowering the incidence of RAO compared with the standard patent hemostasis protocol alone.

Treatment

A. Patients with RAO frequently complain of nonspecific local symptoms, such as pain likely caused by inflammation as a result of instrumentation and/or presence of thrombus. Local therapeutic measures, such as application of cold or hot compresses, and if necessary, a short course of anti-inflammatory agents are usually sufficient in providing relief.

B. Local exercises, such as opening and closing of the hand, exercising the palmar apparatus, flexing and extending the wrist joint, as well as the elbow and the shoulder joints, are frequently effective in relieving the nonspecific symptoms.

C. Recanalization of the radial artery that has been occluded as a result of TRA should not be performed as a default strategy. RAO typically does not cause ischemia in view of extensive collateralization of forearm arterial circulation, and instrumentation is associated with the risk of distal embolization; hence, the potential minor benefit does not justify the risk of distal embolization-related irreversible ischemic consequences.

D. If prophylactic ipsilateral ulnar artery compression was not used during radial hemostatic compression, upon detection of RAO after removal of the radial hemostatic compression device, ipsilateral ulnar compression could be applied to improve the probability of recanalization of RAO before discharge.[16]

E. Systemic anticoagulant therapy could be used in patients who develop RAO to promote recanalization; however, careful weighing of risk versus benefit of systemic anticoagulation, especially keeping major bleeding in mind, is necessary before prescribing such treatment.[27]

RADIAL ARTERITIS

Tenderness along the course of the radial artery with associated localized pain in the absence of RAO is reported by a minority of patients after TRA. This is presumed to be from local inflammation of the radial artery architecture due to instrumentation. It frequently responds to local symptomatically driven treatments, such as cold or warm compresses, and if necessary, anti-inflammatory therapy, including nonsteroidal agents or a short course of corticosteroids. In most instances, it is self-limiting and does not require dedicated treatment.

NONINCLUSIVE RADIAL ARTERY INJURY

Injury to the radial artery wall is very common as shown by elegant studies performed using microscopy,[28] optical coherence tomography, and high-resolution ultrasound,[29–31] although appears to be well tolerated with most patients undergoing TRA not developing any major adverse consequence. Intimal thickening, hypertrophy of the media, as well as increased fibrous burden have been reported. Although not impeding reaccess or hand function, these changes might be of relevance especially if multiple entries are made in the same radial artery over the patient's lifetime.

SUMMARY

Although infrequent, several TRA site-related complications occur in clinical practice. By understanding potential mechanisms related to these complications, several prevention and treatment strategies can be implemented to mitigate adverse outcomes.

REFERENCES

1. Bertrand OF, Bélisle P, Joyal D, et al. Comparison of transradial and femoral approaches for percutaneous coronary interventions: a systematic review and hierarchical Bayesian meta-analysis. Am Heart J 2012;163(4):632–48.
2. He GW, Yang CQ. Characteristics of adrenoceptors in the human radial artery: clinical implications. J Thorac Cardiovasc Surg 1998;115(5):1136–41.
3. Dehghani P, Mohammad A, Bajaj R, et al. Mechanism and predictors of failed transradial approach for percutaneous coronary interventions. JACC Cardiovasc Interv 2009;2(11):1057–64.
4. Seto AH, Roberts JS, Abu-Fadel MS, et al. Real-time ultrasound guidance facilitates transradial access: RAUST (Radial Artery access with Ultrasound Trial). JACC Cardiovasc Interv 2015;8(2):283–91.
5. Pancholy SB, Sanghvi KA, Patel TM. Radial artery access technique evaluation trial: randomized comparison of Seldinger versus modified Seldinger technique for arterial access for transradial catheterization. Catheter Cardiovasc Interv 2012;80(2):288–91.
6. Pancholy SB, Coppola J, Patel T. Subcutaneous administration of nitroglycerin to facilitate radial artery cannulation. Catheter Cardiovasc Interv 2006;68(3):389–91.
7. Rathore S, Stables RH, Pauriah M, et al. Impact of length and hydrophilic coating of the introducer sheath on radial artery spasm during transradial coronary intervention: a randomized study. JACC Cardiovasc Interv 2010;3(5):475–83.
8. Goldsmit A, Kiemeneij F, Gilchrist IC, et al. Radial artery spasm associated with transradial cardiovascular procedures: results from the RAS registry. Catheter Cardiovasc Interv 2014;83(1):E32–6.
9. Patel T, Shah S, Pancholy S. Balloon-assisted tracking of a guide catheter through difficult radial anatomy: a technical report. Catheter Cardiovasc Interv 2013;81(5):E215–8.
10. Koutouzis M, Kontopodis E, Tassopoulos A, et al. Hand hematoma after cardiac catheterization via distal radial artery. J Invasive Cardiol 2018;30(11):428.
11. Bertrand OF. Acute forearm muscle swelling post transradial catheterization and compartment syndrome: prevention is better than treatment! Catheter Cardiovasc Interv 2010;75:366–8.
12. Pancholy SB, Karuparthi PR, Gulati R. A novel nonpharmacologic technique to remove entrapped radial sheath. Catheter Cardiovasc Interv 2015;85(1):E35–8.
13. Mouawad NJ, Capers Q 4th, Allen C, et al. Complete "in situ" avulsion of the radial artery complicating transradial coronary rotational atherectomy. Ann Vasc Surg 2015;29(1):123.e7-11.
14. Zegrı I, Garcıa-Touchard A, Cuenca S, et al. Radial artery pseudoaneurysm following cardiac catheterization: clinical features and nonsurgical treatment results. Rev Esp Cardiol (Engl Ed) 2015;68:349–51.
15. Babunashvili AM, Pancholy SB, Kartashov DS. New technique for treatment of postcatheterization radial artery pseudoaneurysm. Catheter Cardiovasc Interv 2017;89(3):393–8.
16. Bernat I, Bertrand OF, Rokyta R, et al. Efficacy and safety of transient ulnar artery compression to recanalize acute radial artery occlusion after transradial catheterization. Am J Cardiol 2011;107:1698–701.
17. Hahalis GN, Leopoulou M, Tsigkas G, et al. Multicenter randomized evaluation of high versus standard heparin dose on incident radial arterial occlusion after transradial coronary angiography: the SPIRIT OF ARTEMIS Study. JACC Cardiovasc Interv 2018;11(22):2241–50.
18. Plante S, Cantor WJ, Goldman L, et al. Comparison of bivalirudin versus heparin on radial artery occlusion after transradial catheterization. Catheter Cardiovasc Interv 2010;76:654–8.

19. Sanmartin M, Gomez M, Rumoroso JR, et al. Interruption of blood flow during compression and radial artery occlusion after transradial catheterization. Catheter Cardiovasc Interv 2007;70:185–9.

20. Pancholy S, Coppola J, Patel T, et al. Prevention of radial artery occlusion—patent hemostasis evaluation trial (PROPHET study): a randomized comparison of traditional versus patency documented hemostasis after transradial catheterization. Catheter Cardiovasc Interv 2008;72:335–40.

21. Pancholy SB, Patel TM. Effect of duration of hemostatic compression on radial artery occlusion after transradial access. Catheter Cardiovasc Interv 2012;79:78–81.

22. Dangoisse V, Guedès A, Chenu P, et al. Usefulness of a gentle and short hemostasis using the transradial band device after transradial access for percutaneous coronary angiography and interventions to reduce the radial artery occlusion rate (from the prospective and randomized CRASOC I, II, and III studies). Am J Cardiol 2017;120:374–9.

23. Lavi S, Cheema A, Yadegari A, et al. Randomized trial of compression duration after transradial cardiac catheterization and intervention. J Am Heart Assoc 2017;6(2) [pii:e005029].

24. Pancholy SB, Heck LA, Patel T. Forearm arterial anatomy and flow characteristics: a prospective observational study. J Invasive Cardiol 2015;27: 218–21.

25. Koutouzis MJ, Maniotis CD, Avdikos G, et al. ULnar artery transient compression facilitating radial artery patent hemostasis (ULTRA): a novel technique to reduce radial artery occlusion after transradial coronary catheterization. J Invasive Cardiol 2016;28(11):451–4.

26. Pancholy SB, Bernat I, Bertrand OF, et al. Prevention of radial artery occlusion after transradial catheterization: the PROPHET-II randomized trial. JACC Cardiovasc Interv 2016;9:1992–9.

27. Uhlemann M, Gielen S, Woitek FJ, et al. Impact of low molecular weight heparin on reperfusion rates in patients with radial artery occlusion after cardiac catheterization. Results and follow-up in 113 patients. J Am Coll Cardiol 2011;58: B143.

28. Staniloae CS, Mody KP, Sanghvi K, et al. Histopathologic changes of the radial artery wall secondary to transradial catheterization. Vasc Health Risk Manag 2009;5:527–32.

29. Wakeyama T, Ogawa H, Iida H, et al. Intima-media thickening of the radial artery after transradial intervention: an intravascular ultrasound study. J Am Coll Cardiol 2003;41:1109–14.

30. Edmundson A, Mann T. Nonocclusive radial artery injury resulting from transradial coronary interventions: radial artery IVUS. J Invasive Cardiol 2005; 17:528–31.

31. Yonetsu T, Kakuta T, Lee T, et al. Assessment of acute injuries and chronic intimal thickening of the radial artery after transradial coronary intervention by optical coherence tomography. Eur Heart J 2010;31:1608–15.

Optimizing Transradial Access

Radiation, Contrast, Access Site Crossover, and Ergonomics

Jordan G. Safirstein, MD

KEYWORDS

• Transradial • Radiation • Contrast • Ergonomics • Vascular access

KEY POINTS

- Transradial access has been associated with increased radiation exposure, particularly to operators, compared with transfemoral coronary angiography.
- Operator experience, proper shielding, decreasing frame rates, and adjunctive tools may help mitigate radiation exposure.
- Contrast volume is similar between transfemoral and transradial approaches.
- Age of the patient and operator experience are the two strongest predictors of access site crossover.
- The cardiac catheterization laboratory poses significant occupational hazards beyond the radiation, including joint and spine problems.

INTRODUCTION

It has been 3 decades since Campeau[1] published the first series of 100 transradial cardiac catheterizations and since that time the procedure has spread across the world and continues to grow more each year. Along with growth, there must come improvements in efficiency and safety. This article summarizes the data comparing radiation exposures. It focuses on important features that may predict access site failure and crossover and defines the concept of ergonomics in the catheterization laboratory and how clinicians can continue to make their work environments safer and more productive spaces for patients, staff, and physicians.

RADIATION EXPOSURE AND TRANSRADIAL CARDIAC CATHETERIZATION

Scope of Problem

For more than a century, physicians have used ionizing radiation for diagnostic purposes. The widespread availability of radiographs and fluoroscopic imaging has resulted in a dramatic increase in the population's cumulative radiation exposure. X-rays have recently been classified as a carcinogen by the World Health Organization's International Agency for Research on Cancer,[2] and prior reports have suggested that medical exposure may be responsible for as much as 1% of malignancy in the United States.[3] To further frame the use of radiation, the current collective annual dose estimate from medical exposure in the United States has been estimated as roughly similar to the total worldwide collective dose generated by the catastrophe at Chernobyl.[4]

Although interventional cardiac procedures account for only 12% of all radiological studies, they are responsible for delivering the highest radiation dose, accounting for up to 50% of the total collective effective dose.[5] Not until 2010, when the American College of Cardiology (ACC) president called for guidance on appropriate and optimal use of radiation safety

Department of Cardiology, Transradial Intervention, Morristown Medical Center, Meade Level B, 100 Madison Avenue, Morristown, NJ 07960, USA
E-mail address: Jsaf237@yahoo.com

Intervent Cardiol Clin 9 (2020) 99–105
https://doi.org/10.1016/j.iccl.2019.08.001
2211-7458/20/© 2019 Elsevier Inc. All rights reserved.

techniques, were these concerns lauded widely.[6] To this day, many interventionalists still consider radiation protection a perfunctory chore mandated by supervisory committees. However, as the frequency and complexity of interventional cardiac procedures has increased,[7] abundant data regarding increasing stochastic and deterministic risks have surfaced. Reports of increased head and neck cancers,[8] as well as multiple studies indicating at least a 2-fold risk of posterior cataracts,[9] has rallied efforts to protect catheterization laboratory operators and staff.

Radiation exposure to patients is monitored for similar stochastic and deterministic risks using metrics such as fluoroscopy time, cine time, dose area product (DAP), and effective dose. In general, patient exposure is influenced by many factors, including the radiograph equipment performance, protocol used (eg, frame rate), tube angulation, operator experience, and vascular access site.[10]

Radiation Exposure in Transradial Versus Transfemoral Coronary Angiography and Intervention

The transradial approach (TRA) to cardiac catheterization has gained traction in the United States, and across the world, because of its myriad benefits to patients. In addition to fewer vascular complications, decreased bleeding, and a mortality benefit in ST-segment elevation myocardial infarction (STEMI), patients prefer TRA, ambulate faster, and are discharged sooner than with the transfemoral approach (TFA) to cardiac catheterization. Furthermore, recent studies have shown significant cost savings with the use of TRA rather than TFA to facilitate same-day discharge.[11,12] Despite these advantages and its continued growth, TRA is a technically more demanding procedure with a well-described learning curve, and still contends with increased radiation exposure to both patients and operators as a persistent safety issue compared with TFA.[13]

Radiation exposure of TRA compared with TFA has been extensively studied, with randomized trials first reported in 2008.[14,15] Numerous randomized and observational studies comparing access sites have consistently shown increased operator exposure associated with the radial approach. However, there is some evidence suggesting that operator experience may improve operator exposure over time. Bundhoo and colleagues[16] retrospectively analyzed a single-center transition from mostly TFA to greater than 90% TRA over 5 years, and showed comparable fluoroscopy time and radiation dose once an operator performed more than 60% of the procedures radially. Subsequently, Becher and colleagues[17] prospectively evaluated 400 patients, showing no difference in fluoroscopy time, procedural duration, radiation dose, or contrast use between TRA and TFA in percutaneous coronary intervention (PCI). In addition, Jolly and colleagues[18] reported in a substudy of the RIVAL (Radial versus femoral access for coronary angiography and intervention in patients with acute coronary syndromes) trial that the nominal increase in air kerma associated with TRA was only present in lower-volume centers and operators, supporting the hypothesis that experience mitigates radiation exposure. Plourde and colleagues[19] showed similar experience-driven improvements in radiation exposure in transfemoral procedures as well. It is important to recognize that operator exposure in these trials used fluoroscopy time and/or DAP as their metrics of operator exposure, as opposed to dosimetry, the gold standard for measuring operator exposure.

Even in spite of operator proficiency, there are subsets of patients in whom operators, regardless of experience, have been shown to have higher radiation exposure. In a prospective study of 128 patients that had undergone coronary artery bypass graft surgery, Michael and colleagues[20] showed that TRA for diagnostic coronary angiography yielded longer procedure times, greater patient air kerma radiation exposure, and higher operator dose compared with TFA. Casting further controversy on the concept of experience mitigating operator exposure is the most recent (and largest) randomized trial to date, the RAD-MATRIX (RAdiation Dose study - Minimizing Adverse Haemorrhagic Events by TRansradial Access Site and Systemic Implementation of angioX) trial. Sciahbhasi and colleagues[21] used individual dosimeters at wrist, thorax, and head to directly measure operator exposure in 8404 patients randomized to the TRA or TFA approach, who were undergoing coronary angiography and percutaneous intervention in patients with or without STEMI. Even in experienced radial operators (those performing >100 TRA procedures per year), operator exposure (measured in the most direct method available) was significantly higher with TRA compared with TFA. Radial procedures were associated with a near-double increase in radiation burden at the chest level, as measured by a dedicated dosimeter worn outside the breast pocket. Patient radiation exposure was also significantly higher, but to a lesser degree.

Radiation Exposure in Left Versus Right Radial Approach

Although some studies have shown lower radiation exposure from the left radial approach (LRA) versus right radial approach (RRA), others find no difference, and 1 showed that RRA was associated with lower radiation exposure than LRA.[22–25] Given the more complex anatomic pathway from the RRA, increased fluoroscopy time and DAP logically follow. One study did show increased radiation exposure from the LRA, which may be attributable to a shorter distance to scatter radiation working from the right side of the patient, or possibly, given that most operators work much more often from the right side, unfamiliarity may breed less efficiency and more need for fluoroscopic imaging.[26] Data from the RAD-MATRIX trial contribute further to the conflicting reports regarding LRA versus RRA, showing no difference in patient or operator radiation exposure between the two approaches.

Techniques to Decrease Radiation Exposure During Transradial Coronary Angiography and Intervention

Understanding why radiation exposure to the operator is consistently higher with TRA is essential to resolving the issue, and several potential reasons exist:

- The transition from the subclavian to ascending aorta demands consistent fluoroscopic visualization, unlike the relatively straightforward ascension up the aorta.
- The tortuosity of the right innominate-aortic system often requires maneuvers involving deep breaths and use of floppy, hydrophilic, or very stiff wires that add additional fluoroscopic imaging that TFA rarely requires.
- Variable arm positioning for TRA and patient setup frequently result in an operator closer to the radiation source than would be needed with TFA.
- Because of the need for access to the arterial sheath in the wrist, shielding often rests closer to the patient, resulting in less efficient protection against scatter radiation.

Acknowledging and accepting the increased radiation burden of TRA should prompt simple and effective interventions, such as usage of a larger upper shield and adducting the arm closer to the body to significantly reduce exposure to the operator, as shown in the RAD-MATRIX trial. Other recent introductions to the safety armamentarium include affordable lead and bismuth drapes (eg, Radpad), which have shown the ability to significantly reduce exposure to the operator by as much as 23%.[27] Recent studies have also shown that operator and patient radiation exposure can be markedly reduced by decreasing frame rates and using selective storage of fluoroscopic images,[28] without diminishing the quality of the angiogram.[29,30] In addition, appropriate use of collimation and attention to proper positioning of the image intensifier yield significant reductions in radiation exposure to the operator.

The literature on radiation exposure is young but has provided the cardiology community with important knowledge with which to improve. Recognizing that TRA may be associated with increased radiation exposure, particularly to operators, should prompt institutions to implement the use of proper shielding techniques, aggressive monitoring of patients and operators, use of adjunctive devices, and changes in protocols that foster a safer and healthier catheterization laboratory.

CONTRAST USE IN TRANSRADIAL VERSUS TRANSFEMORAL CORONARY ANGIOGRAPHY AND INTERVENTION

Contrast use during cardiac catheterization is an important topic because there is a direct, dose-dependent relationship between contrast volume and postprocedural acute kidney injury (AKI), specifically, contrast-induced nephropathy (CIN).[31] CIN has been associated with increased in-hospital mortality and worse long-term outcomes.[32] Although there have been trials showing larger volumes of contrast with TRA,[20,33] more recent reports have shown equivocal or less contrast use with TRA.[21,34] A recent meta-analysis reviewing 13 randomized controlled trials, all of which included experienced radial operators, showed no significant difference in contrast volume between radial and femoral approaches.[35] Of note, the trials showing higher contrast volumes were comparing TRA with TFA for octogenarians and patients with coronary artery bypass grafts, both population subsets in which TRA is known to be more challenging.

A retrospective analysis of nearly 230,000 patients with chronic kidney disease, within the Veterans' Affairs health system, undergoing cardiac catheterization found that TRA was associated with lower risk for both postprocedure transfusion and progression to end-stage renal disease at 1 year, compared with TFA.[36] The randomized RAD-MATRIX trial showed a lower rate of AKI with TRA (15.4%) versus TFA (17.4%).[21] These findings may be a result of avoiding the atheromatous aorta and renal vessels, thereby lessening the chance of atheroembolization. Alternatively, TRA also has the known benefit of less frequent transfusions and bleeding complications, both independent predictors of AKI.[37,38]

ACCESS SITE CROSSOVER DURING TRANSRADIAL ACCESS

The radial approach continues to grow in prevalence in the United States year after year. However, TRA PCI still accounts for just 37% of all interventions according to the American College of Cardiology's National Cardiovascular Data Registry (ACC-NCDR), which is consistent growth but far from the dominant strategy.[39] Multiple anatomic and technical challenges of TRA exist that steepen the initial learning curve, contribute to its higher rate of access site crossover compared with TFA, and limit its widespread adoption.

Access site failure poses additional challenges to patients and operators in as much as it results in longer procedural times, increased fluoroscopy time and radiation exposure to both patients and operators, and adds the additional risk of a second arterial puncture. Le and colleagues[40] retrospectively reviewed 1600 procedures performed at a single center to identify patient and procedural characteristics that predict crossover from TRA to TFA. Overall, the study reported a 10.4% crossover rate, with operators that had less than 5 years' experience faring significantly worse than their experienced colleagues (13.2% vs 5.2% crossover rate). Importantly, access site crossover in those with less TRA experience decreased over time as operator use of TRA increased. randomized controlled trials that included experienced operators have reported access site crossover rates ranging from 3% to 7%,[41,42] and multiple other studies have shown lack of operator experience as a predictor of crossover.[43] Although operator experience may be a modifiable factor, LRA has been shown to confront significantly less subclavian tortuosity and may be a better option for new operators.[22,44] As described earlier, most cardiac catheterization laboratories are designed to work from the right side of the

patient, making the LRA an undesirable and often uncomfortable access choice for most operators.

Multiple investigators have similarly found age to be predictive of TRA failure, including Dehghani and colleagues,[45] who performed a large retrospective study and reported that age more than 75 years and short stature, as well as prior coronary artery bypass graft surgery, were associated with TRA failure. Other studies have found that female gender, short stature, hypertension, and high body mass index are associated with severe subclavian tortuosity, and hence increased risk of TRA failure.[46] Operators may consider using LRA rather than RRA in patients with these characteristics.

ERGONOMIC CONSIDERATIONS OF THE TRANSRADIAL APPROACH

Ergonomics is the study of people in their working environments with the goal of improving efficiency, eliminating discomfort, and minimizing risk of injury. In the cardiac catheterization laboratory, there are a multitude of ergonomic challenges that confront all staff who participate in fluoroscopy-guided procedures. Protective lead garments weigh heavily on joints and spine; radiation exposure is an ever-present concern; and lifting, supporting, and transferring patients is physically taxing.

Klein and colleagues[47] surveyed 314 members of the Society of Cardiac Angiography and Intervention and found that 49% of respondents reported at least 1 orthopedic injury related to their occupation. Annual total caseload was directly related to prevalence of orthopedic injury. However, these physical stresses are likely caused by protective apparel that shields operators from radiation injury. In a subsequent study, survey responses from 1042 catheterization laboratory workers and 499 controls (those not exposed to radiation) revealed that those wearing protective lead garments were more likely to have work-related pain, and to have sought medical care for it, than the control group. They were also more likely to report pain at the time of the survey. The association between work-related pain and lead apron wearing remained after adjustment for age, sex, body mass index, preexisting musculoskeletal conditions, years in the profession, and job description (adjusted odds ratio, 1.67; 95% confidence interval, 1.32–2.11).[48]

Ergonomic interventions may include simple and effective strategies such as using the lightest protective lead possible, with lumbar support, and wearing comfortable footwear and compression stockings. More complex ergonomic interventions, such as Zero Gravity, is a ceiling-suspended lead shield that allows the operators to work completely protected but without the heavy burden of lead weighing them down. Robotic PCI goes 1 step further by permitting operators to work in a comfortably seated position, behind leaded glass, from across the room, or even further afield.[49]

In order to prevent work-related musculoskeletal injury in the catheterization laboratory, there needs to be cooperation between those inside the catheterization laboratory and those who manage it. All members of the team, from the housekeeping crew to the director, should be encouraged to identify ergonomic issues, implement solutions, and evaluate their progress.

Although TRA has grown steadily, most cases are done from the right side, most likely as a result of operator comfort, room design, and staff convenience. Kado and colleagues[50] randomized 100 patients to LRA or RRA and found that although radiation exposure was significantly higher from the RRA, more operator discomfort was reported with LRA access. Setup of LRA patients is a unique challenge and setup may vary between institutions and even operators within the same institution. Preparation of LRA patients may involve arm slings, eye drapes, various clamps, and an array of towels to preserve sterility. Although LRA has advantages for the operator (less tortuosity, better shielding, decreased operator exposure), the lack of a standardized and dependable setup in most catheterization laboratories produces an insurmountable ergonomic challenge.

Several recent advances in LRA procedures may have a major impact on the ability to standardize the setup process and make the procedure more comfortable for staff and operators. Recent additions to the armamentarium include specifically designed arm boards (Cobra Board by TZ Medical; STARBoard by Adept) made to elevate and buttress the left arm, preventing the drift that otherwise occurs during the procedure. Alternatively (and less expensively), our laboratory uses a 30° wedge to angle the patient toward the right side of the table, as well as an arm sling to support the wrist throughout the procedure.

The distal radial, or snuff box, approach allows the patient's left arm to be comfortably pronated and placed on the abdomen, flexed at a 45° angle at the elbow, allowing for a comfortable access position for the operator from either side of the table. Limited available data thus far have shown comparable rates of vascular complications, radial artery occlusion, and procedural success.[51]

SUMMARY

In order to ensure a safe experience for both patients and physicians, clinicians must continue to evaluate and adjust how they perform transradial cardiac catheterization. As procedures become more complex and more percutaneous solutions become available, the onus is on the interventional community to remain vigilant about making their work environment safe for all. Diminishing radiation exposure, minimizing contrast use, preventing access site failure, and creating the healthiest possible work environment will ensure that transradial intervention continues to flourish for years to come.

REFERENCES

1. Campeau L. Percutaneous radial artery approach for coronary angiography. Cathet Cardiovasc Diagn 1989;16(1):3–7.
2. Amis ES, Butler PF, Applegate KE. American College of Radiology white paper on radiation dose in medicine. J Am Coll Radiol 2007;4:272–84.
3. Berrington de Gonzalez A, Darby S. Risk of cancer from diagnostic x-rays: estimates for the UK and 14 other countries. Lancet 2004;363:345–51.
4. Annex D. Exposures from the chernobyl accident. UNSCEAR report; 1988. Available at: http://www.unscear.org/docs/reports/1988annexd.pdf.
5. Picano E, Vano E, Semelka R, et al. The American College of Radiology white paper on radiation dose in medicine: deep impact on the practice of cardiovascular imaging. Cardiovasc Ultrasound 2007;5:37.
6. Brindis R, Douglas PS. President's page: the ACC encourages multi-pronged approach to radiation safety. J Am Coll Cardiol 2010;56(6):522–4.
7. Cousins C, Miller DL, Bernardi G, et al. ICRP publication 120: radiological protection in cardiology. Ann ICRP 2013;42:1–125.
8. Roguin A, Goldstein J, Bar O, et al. Brain and neck tumors among physicians performing interventional procedures. Am J Cardiol 2013;111(9):1368–72.
9. Ciraj-Bjelac O, Rehani M, Minamoto AA, et al. Radiation-induced eye lens changes and risk for cataract in interventional cardiology. Cardiology 2012; 123:168–71.
10. Tsapaki V, Kottou S, Vano E, et al. Patient dose values in a dedicated Greek cardiac centre. Br J Radiol 2003;76(910):726–30.
11. Agostoni P, Biondi-Zoccai GG, de Benedictis ML, et al. Radial versus femoral approach for

percutaneous coronary diagnostic and interventional procedures; systematic overview and meta-analysis of randomized trials. J Am Coll Cardiol 2004;44:349–56.

12. Amin AP, House JA, Safley DM, et al. Costs of transradial percutaneous coronary intervention. JACC Cardiovasc Interv 2013;6:827–34.

13. Ball WT, Sharieff W, Jolly SS, et al. Characterization of operator learning curve for transradial coronary interventions. Circ Cardiovasc Interv 2011;4:336–41.

14. Brasselet C, Blanpain T, Tassan-Mangina S, et al. Comparison of operator radiation exposure with optimized radiation protection devices during coronary angiograms and ad hoc percutaneous coronary interventions by radial and femoral routes. Eur Heart J 2008;29:63–70.

15. Brueck M, Bandorski D, Kramer W, et al. A randomized comparison of transradial versus transfemoral approach for coronary angiography and angioplasty. JACC Cardiovasc Interv 2009;2:1047–54.

16. Bundhoo S, Nallur-Shivu G, Ossei-Gerning N, et al. Switching from transfemoral to transradial access for PCI: a single-center learning curve over 5 years. J Invasive Cardiol 2014;26:535–41.

17. Becher T, Behnes M, Unsal M, et al. Radiation exposure and contrast agent use related to radial versus femoral arterial access during percutaneous coronary intervention (PCI)—results of the FERARI Study. Cardiovasc Revasc Med 2016;17(8):505–9.

18. Jolly SS, Cairns J, Niemela K, et al. Effect of radial versus femoral access on radiation dose and the importance of procedural volume: a substudy of the multicenter randomized RIVAL trial. JACC Cardiovasc Interv 2013;6:258–66.

19. Plourde G, Pancholy SB, Nolan J, et al. Radiation exposure in relation to the arterial access site used for diagnostic coronary angiography and percutaneous coronary intervention: a systematic review and meta-analysis. Lancet 2015;386:2192–203.

20. Michael TT, Alomar M, Papayannis A, et al. A randomized comparison of the transradial and transfemoral approaches for coronary artery bypass graft angiography and intervention: the RADIAL-CABG Trial (RADIAL Versus Femoral Access for Coronary Artery Bypass Graft Angiography and Intervention). JACC Cardiovasc Interv 2013;6:1138–44.

21. Sciahbasi A, Frigoli E, Sarandrea A, et al. Radiation exposure and vascular access in acute coronary syndromes: the RAD-matrix trial. J Am Coll Cardiol 2017;69(20):2530–7.

22. Sciahbasi A, Romagnoli E, Burzotta F, et al. Transradial approach (left vs right) and procedural times during percutaneous coronary procedures: TALENT Study. Am Heart J 2011;161:172–9.

23. Hu H, Fu Q, Chen W, et al. A prospective randomized comparison of left and right radial approach for percutaneous coronary angiography in Asian populations. Clin Interv Aging 2014;9:963–8.

24. Dominici M, Diletti R, Milici C, et al. Left radial versus right radial approach for coronary artery catheterization: a prospective comparison. J Interv Cardiol 2012;25:203–9.

25. Guo X, Ding J, Qi Y, et al. Left radial access is preferable to right radial access for the diagnostic or interventional coronary procedures: a meta-analysis involving 22 randomized clinical trials and 10287 patients. PLoS One 2013;8:e78499.

26. Pancholy S, Joshi P, Shah S, et al. Effect of vascular access site choice on radiation exposure during coronary angiography. JACC Cardiovasc Interv 2015;8(9):1189–96.

27. Vlastra W, Delewi R, Sjauw KD, et al. Efficacy of the RADPAD protection drape in reducing operators' radiation exposure in the catheterization laboratory: a sham-controlled randomized trial. Circ Cardiovasc Interv 2017;10(11) [pii:e006058].

28. Shah B, Mai X, Tummala L, et al. Effectiveness of fluorography versus cineangiography at reducing radiation exposure during diagnostic coronary angiography. Am J Cardiol 2014;113(7):1093–8.

29. Maccagni D, Candilio L, Latib A, et al. Implementation of a low frame-rate protocol and noise-reduction technology to minimize radiation dose in transcatheter aortic valve replacement. J Invasive Cardiol 2018;30(5):169–75.

30. Chon MK, Chun KJ, Lee DS, et al. Radiation reduction during percutaneous coronary intervention: a new protocol with a low frame rate and selective fluoroscopic image storage. Medicine (Baltimore) 2017;96(30):e7517.

31. Mehran R, Aymong ED, Nikolsky E, et al. A simple risk score for prediction of contrast-induced nephropathy after percutaneous coronary intervention: development and initial validation. J Am Coll Cardiol 2004;44:1393–9.

32. Rihal CS, Textor SC, Grill DE, et al. Incidence and prognostic importance of acute renal failure after percutaneous coronary intervention. Circulation 2002;105:2259–64.

33. Jaffe R, Hong T, Sharieff W, et al. Comparison of radial versus femoral approach for percutaneous coronary interventions in octogenarians. Catheter Cardiovasc Interv 2007;69:815–20.

34. Andò G, Cortese B, Russo F, et al, MATRIX Investigators. Acute kidney injury after radial or femoral access for invasive acute coronary syndrome management: AKI-MATRIX. J Am Coll Cardiol 2017. [Epub ahead of print].

35. Shah R, Mattox A, Khan MR, et al. Contrast use in relation to the arterial access site for percutaneous coronary intervention: a comprehensive meta-analysis of randomized trials. World J Cardiol 2017;9(4):378–83.

36. Vora A, Stanislawski M, Grunwald G, et al. Association Between Chronic Kidney Disease and rates of transfusion and progression to end-stage renal disease in patients undergoing transradial versus transfemoral cardiac catheterization—an analysis from the Veterans Affairs Clinical Assessment Reporting and Tracking (CART) program. J Am Heart Assoc 2017;6(4) [pii:e004819].

37. Ohno Y, Maekawa Y, Miyata H, et al. Impact of periprocedural bleeding on incidence of contrast-induced acute kidney injury in patients treated with percutaneous coronary intervention. J Am Coll Cardiol 2013;62:1260–6.

38. Roy P, Raya V, Okabe T, et al. Incidence, predictors, and outcomes of post-percutaneous coronary intervention nephropathy in patients with diabetes mellitus and normal baseline serum creatinine levels. Am J Cardiol 2008;101:1544–9.

39. Waldo S, Gokhale M, O'Donnell C, et al. Temporal trends in coronary angiography and percutaneous coronary intervention: insights from the VA clinical assessment, reporting, and tracking program. JACC Cardiovasc Interv 2018;11(9): 879–88.

40. Le J, Bangalore S, Guo Y, et al. Predictors of access site crossover in patients who underwent transradial coronary angiography. Am J Cardiol 2015; 116(3):379–83.

41. Ratib K, Mamas MA, Anderson SG, et al, British Cardiovascular Intervention Society and the National Institute for Cardiovascular Outcomes Research. Access site practice and procedural outcomes in relation to clinical presentation in 439,947 patients undergoing percutaneous coronary intervention in the United kingdom. JACC Cardiovasc Interv 2015;8(pt A):20–9.

42. Romagnoli E, Biondi-Zoccai G, Sciahbasi A, et al. Radial versus femoral randomized investigation in ST-segment elevation acute coronary syndrome: the RIFLE-STEACS (Radial Versus Femoral Randomized Investigation in ST-Elevation Acute Coronary Syndrome) study. J Am Coll Cardiol 2012;60:2481–9.

43. Rubartelli P, Crimi G, Bartolini D, et al. Switching from femoral to routine radial access site for ST-elevation myocardial infarction: a single center experience. J Interv Cardiol 2014;27:591–9.

44. Burzotta F, Trani C, Mazzari MA, et al. Vascular complications and access crossover in 10,676 transradial percutaneous coronary procedures. Am Heart J 2012;163:230–8.

45. Dehghani P, Mohammad A, Bajaj R, et al. Mechanism and Predictors of Failed Transradial Approach for Percutaneous Coronary Interventions. JACC Cardiovasc Interv 2009;2(11):1057–64.

46. Abdelaal E, Brousseau-Provencher C, Montminy S, et al. Risk score, causes, and clinical impact of failure of transradial approach for percutaneous coronary interventions. JACC Cardiovasc Interv 2013; 6(11):1129–37.

47. Klein LW, Miller DL, Balter S, et al. Occupational health hazards in the interventional laboratory: time for a safer environment. Catheter Cardiovasc Interv 2018. [Epub ahead of print].

48. Orme NM, Rihal CS, Gulati R, et al. Occupational health hazards of working in the interventional laboratory: a multisite case control study of physicians and allied staff. J Am Coll Cardiol 2015;65:820–6.

49. Weisz G, Metzger DC, Caputo RP, et al. Safety and feasibility of robotic percutaneous coronary intervention: PRECISE (Percutaneous Robotically-Enhanced Coronary Intervention) Study. J Am Coll Cardiol 2013;61(15):1596–600.

50. Kado H, Patel AM, Suryadevara S, et al. Operator radiation exposure and physical discomfort during a right versus left radial approach for coronary interventions: a randomized evaluation. JACC Cardiovasc Interv 2014;7(7):810–6.

51. Kiemeneij F. Left distal transradial access in the anatomical snuffbox for coronary angiography (ldTRA) and interventions (ldTRI). EuroIntervention 2017;13(7):851–7.

The Value of Transradial

Impact on Patient Satisfaction and Health Care Economics

Samuel M. Lindner, MD[a,b], Christian A. McNeely, MD[a,b],
Amit P. Amin, MD, MSc[a,b,c,*]

KEYWORDS

- Transradial versus femoral access • Transradial approach • Cardiac catheterization

KEY POINTS

- Transradial access improves clinical outcomes, primarily through decreased bleeding and vascular access site complications, and has demonstrated a mortality benefit in patients with acute coronary syndromes.
- In surveys, patients report a preference for transradial over transfemoral access for cardiac catheterization because of greater overall comfort, less pain, and decreased ambulatory impairment.
- Transradial access offers cost savings over transfemoral access, primarily through decreased length of stay, reduced resource utilization, and reduced rates of complications.
- Transradial access facilitates same-day discharge, leading to increased patient satisfaction and better health care value, particularly in an era of alternative payment models and bundled payments.

INTRODUCTION

Transradial access (TRA) for diagnostic coronary angiography and percutaneous coronary intervention (PCI) has been used in clinical practice for more than 25 years.[1,2] Early techniques for coronary angiography via the Sones technique used brachial artery cutdown access and required specialized training for proficiency, but development of transfemoral access (TFA) using the Seldinger technique and preformed specialized catheters proved more operator-friendly and led to widespread adoption of TFA as the mainstay for both diagnostic and PCI access for many years.[3–7] In a National Cardiovascular Data Registry (NCDR) analysis of more than 600 procedural centers, radial access accounted for only 1.32% of total PCI procedures from 2004 to 2007.[8] Since then, multiple studies have demonstrated various benefits of TRA over TFA, notably less bleeding, vascular access complications, and cardiovascular events.[9–13] In recent years, there has been a surge in the adoption of TRA for PCI.[14–16] In an updated NCDR analysis examining radial utilization, although TRA was used in only 1.2% of

Disclosures: Dr S.M. Lindner is a consultant to AstraZeneca. C.A. McNeely: None. Dr A.P. Amin is funded via a comparative effectiveness research KM1 Career Development Award from the Clinical and Translational Science Award program of the National Center for Advancing Translational Sciences of the National Institutes of Health, grant numbers UL1TR000448, KL2TR000450, and TL-1TR000449, and the National Cancer Institute of the National Institutes of Health, grant number 1KM1CA156708-01; an AHRQ R18 grant award (grant number R18HS0224181-01A1); and is a consultant to GE HealthCare, Terumo, and AstraZeneca.

[a] Cardiovascular Division, Washington University School of Medicine, 660 S Euclid Avenue, Campus Box 8086, St Louis, MO 63110, USA; [b] Barnes-Jewish Hospital, 660 S Euclid Avenue, Campus Box 8086, St Louis, MO 63110, USA; [c] Center for Value and Innovation, Washington University School of Medicine, 660 S Euclid Avenue, Campus Box 8086, St Louis, MO 63110, USA

* Corresponding author. Cardiovascular Division, Washington University School of Medicine, 660 S Euclid Avenue, Campus Box 8086, St Louis, MO 63110.

E-mail address: aamin@wustl.edu

cases at the beginning of 2007, utilization increased to 16.1% of cases by the end of 2012.[15] This trend has continued, and according to NCDR CathPCI registry institutional report data for 2019, radial access utilization is approaching 40%.[16] Because of mounting data emphasizing the tolerability, safety, and cost-effectiveness of TRA, there has been growing support of a "radial first strategy."[17,18] In this review, the authors discuss the advantages of TRA for patient satisfaction, patient safety, and the economic impact on hospitals and the health care system.

IMPACT ON PATIENT SATISFACTION

Multiple randomized clinical trials comparing radial versus femoral access for angiography or PCI have shown consistent patient preference for radial over femoral access.[10,13,19,20] In the RIVAL trial, which randomized more than 7000 patients, greater than 70% of those surveyed indicated a preference for radial over femoral access for their next procedure (hazard ratio [HR] 8.99, 95% confidence interval [CI] 7.86–10.28; P<.0001).[10] In SAFE-PCI, women undergoing radial access for diagnostic angiography or PCI were more likely to prefer the same access route for their next procedure than women who underwent femoral access (77.2% vs 26.8%; P<.0001), although assessments with validated instruments showed no measurable difference in quality of life in radial versus femoral groups.[13,21] For patients who had undergone both TRA and TFA in the CARAFE study, 58% preferred TRA versus 21% preferred TFA and 21% had no preference.[19] Cooper and colleagues[20] conducted another randomized trial involving 200 patients that also showed the vast majority of patients strongly preferred radial access. Specifically, patients rated radial access as being more comfortable than femoral access, and patients undergoing femoral access reported more associated back pain and difficulty walking.[19,20] Survey data investigating patient preference related to vascular access during cardiac catheterization showed that decreased risk of major bleeding was a top priority for satisfaction, followed by desires for decreased length of stay (LOS) and maximized postprocedural mobilization.[22]

PATIENT SAFETY AND BLEEDING RISK

In randomized trials, TRA has demonstrated lower rates of bleeding, vascular access site complications (VASCs), composite outcomes of major adverse cardiovascular events (MACE),

and net adverse clinical events (NACE).[9–13] In particular, data show safety benefits in the setting of acute coronary syndrome (ACS), when patients are at risk for bleeding complications related to receiving anticoagulation and antiplatelet agents. In targeted analyses of populations at high risk for procedural complications, including women, the elderly, and the severely obese, radial access was shown to improve clinical outcomes.[13,23–25]

In the MATRIX trial, which randomized 8404 patients with ACS to radial or femoral access, investigators observed lower rates of MACE in the TRA group (8.8% vs 10.3%; relative risk [RR] 0.85, 95% CI 0.74–0.99; P = .0307), although this was not a statistically significant finding based on a prespecified α of 0.025. There were also reduced rates of NACE favoring TRA (9.8% vs 11.7%; RR 0.83, 95% CI 0.73–0.96; P = .0092). In the TRA group, there were decreased bleeding rates when taking all major and minor bleeding indices into account (8.4% vs 14.4%; RR 0.55, 95% CI 0.48–0.63; P<.0001). In the TFA group, there were significantly higher access site–related bleeding academic research consortium (BARC) major bleeding, bleeding requiring blood transfusion, and VASC requiring surgical intervention.[9]

Comparatively, the RIVAL trial randomized 7021 patients with ACS to radial or femoral access and found no difference in the primary outcome of composite all-cause mortality, myocardial infarction (MI), stroke, or noncoronary artery bypass surgery (CABG) bleeding at 30 days (3.7% vs 4.0%; HR 0.92, 95% CI 0.72–1.17; P = .5). There was also no difference between the groups in the individual outcomes of death, MI, or stroke. There were significantly lower rates of VASCs in patients undergoing radial compared with femoral intervention (1.4% vs 3.7%, P<.0001). Although there was no statistical difference in primary safety endpoints of non-CABG thrombolysis in myocardial infarction major bleeding, CABG-related bleeding, non-CABG-related blood transfusions, or all blood transfusions between TRA versus TFA, a post hoc exploratory outcome analysis showed TRA was associated with significantly decreased ACUITY major bleeding (defined as non-CABG major bleeding, large hematoma, or pseudoaneurysm requiring repair) when compared with TFA (1.9% vs 4.5%, P<.0001).[10]

In the RIFLE-STEACS trial, 1001 patients with ST-elevation ACS, including those with cardiogenic shock and failed thrombolysis, were randomized to TRA versus TFA for intervention by experienced radial operators (those using radial access in more than 50% of cases). There was a significant reduction in the primary outcome of NACE, defined as the composite of cardiac death, stroke, MI, target lesion revascularization, and bleeding, in the TRA versus TFA group (13.6% vs 21.0%, P = .003). The radial arm showed significantly lower rates of MACE and cardiac death, implying a mortality benefit in ACS patients. Bleeding complications were also lower in the TRA versus TFA arm with hemoglobin drop ≥3 g/dL (6.0% vs 9.8%, P = .036) and bleeding requiring blood transfusion (1.0% vs 3.2%, P = .025). Access site–related bleeding was 2.6% in the radial group versus 6.8% in the femoral group (P = .002). Overall non-CABG-associated bleeding rate was 10% (7.8% in TRA vs 12.2% in TFA, P = .026). Investigators noted that considerable overall bleeding rates may have been partially explained by use of glycoprotein IIb/IIIa in 69% of these patients, which was not uncommon at the time of trial conduct. There was no difference between TRA and TFA groups for the use of these agents, implying that TRA reduces bleeding when these agents are used.[11]

In a similar setting of ST-elevation ACS, 707 patients were randomized to radial versus femoral intervention by experienced operators across 4 high-volume centers in the STEMI-RADIAL trial. Operators were trained in the femoral approach but practiced in high-volume radial centers (centers with >80% radial cases). The TRA group compared with the TFA group demonstrated a significant reduction in the primary outcome of major bleeding or VASCs at 30 days (1.4% vs 7.2%, P = .0001). There was a significant reduction in NACE defined as composite of death, MI, stroke, and major bleeding/vascular complications with TRA versus TFA. This reduction was primarily driven by decreased bleeding, because there was no statistical difference in MACE, MI, stroke, or death. With follow-up at 30 days and 6 months, there was significantly less major bleeding in the radial group (1.4% vs 7.2%, P = .0001), even when vascular closure devices were used in 38% of femoral cases.[12] The investigators noted that a subgroup analysis of the femoral group showed no significant difference in bleeding or VASCs in those who did versus those who did not receive vascular closure. Overall, vascular complication rates were low at 0.6%, and there was no significant difference between radial and femoral groups.[12]

SAFE-PCI, a registry-based randomized trial evaluating the effect of TRA versus TFA on outcomes in women undergoing PCI, enrolled 1787 women referred for urgent or elective PCI or diagnostic catheterization with possible subsequent PCI. Patients having ST-elevation ACS were excluded. Of note, women have smaller radial arteries on average and are a population at higher risk of catheter-related complications. Radial access resulted in a statistically significant 70% reduction in the primary composite endpoint of bleeding or VASCs requiring intervention in patients undergoing diagnostic catheterization or PCI (0.6% vs 1.7%; odds ratio 0.32; 95% CI 0.12–0.90). In patients undergoing PCI, there was a 60% reduction in the primary endpoint, but this was not statistically significant. This trial was stopped early by the data safety and monitoring board because of lower-than-expected event rates.[13]

Overall, randomized trials evaluating TRA versus TFA consistently show fewer complications related to bleeding and vascular access, and these benefits are confirmed in large meta-analyses that demonstrate decreased bleeding and VASCs as well as mortality benefit in the ACS population, with TRA versus TFA.[26,27] Analyses of large registries support these findings.[8,14,16,28] Further insights will follow formal publication of data from the Safety and Efficacy of Femoral Access versus Radial Access in STEMI Trial (SAFARI-STEMI), a randomized trial that compares TRA to TFA in the setting of ST-elevation ACS with high utilization of bivalirudin and vascular closure devices as bleeding-avoidance strategies (NCT01398254).[29] Taken in total, the evidence evaluating outcomes in TRA versus TFA has led to recommendations that a "radial first" strategy may be reasonable to maximize patient safety.[18]

IMPACT ON EARLY AMBULATION AND LENGTH OF STAY

Patients have reported a strong preference for earlier ambulation and decreased LOS.[22] Although the RIVAL trial of more than 7000 randomized patients found no difference in LOS between TRA and TFA arms (4 days vs 4 days, P = .18),[10] multiple subsequent studies have shown that patients undergoing cardiac catheterization and PCI by TRA experienced early ambulation and decreased LOS compared with those performed by TFA. By anatomic location alone, radial access has an advantage over femoral access for early ambulation. Although bed rest times after femoral access may be shortened with the use of vascular closure devices or reduced femoral sheath diameters, this has been shown to increase procedural cost or decrease angiographic quality.[30]

The RADIAMI trial demonstrated that among patients hospitalized with MI, TRA significantly reduced bed rest time by greater than 12 hours compared with TFA (P<.003).[31] Similarly, in the CARAFE study, bed rest times in patients undergoing TRA were halved compared with TFA (4.9 hours vs 9.9 hours, P<.001), and LOS was significantly reduced in TRA versus TFA (31 hours vs 42 hours, P<.05).[19] In a series of elderly patients having elective catheterization, radial access was also associated with earlier ambulation time (5 hours vs 11 hours, P<.001), although LOS was short in both radial and femoral access groups with no significant difference.[32] These findings were confirmed in a metaanalysis of mostly nonrandomized studies and show a consistent benefit in early ambulation favoring radial access over femoral access in elderly patients undergoing cardiac catheterization.[33] The effect of radial access on LOS has also been evaluated in large randomized trials of patients with ACS. In RIFLE-STEACS, patients undergoing TRA had statistically significant decreases in total hospital LOS and LOS in the intensive care unit versus TFA (3 vs 4 days, P<.001).[11] STEMI-RADIAL also showed a significant reduction in intensive care unit LOS in the TRA versus TFA arm (2.5 vs 3.0 days, P = .0038).[12]

These data show that most randomized trials evaluating radial versus femoral access in the setting of ACS demonstrate an advantage in radial access for decreasing time to ambulation and having potential for reduced LOS. In the setting of stable coronary disease and planned outpatient cardiac catheterization, early ambulation with radial access facilitates same-day discharge (SDD) plans and is aligned with patient satisfaction priorities.

IMPLICATIONS FOR HEALTH CARE ECONOMICS

In efforts to motivate improvements in cost efficiency, payers have been exploring alternative payment models as part of a shift in the US health care system from volume-based to value-based reimbursement.[34] The Centers for Medicare and Medicaid's Innovation Bundled Payments for Care Improvement initiative, commonly referred to as "bundled payments," has been continued as a voluntary program to incentivize high-quality, cost-saving care practices.[34,35] Through lower risk of bleeding and VASCs, earlier ambulation, and decreased LOS, TRA results in cost savings and safety benefits for patients, payers, hospitals, and the health care system as a whole. There is evidence of cost advantages in a range of catheterization settings.[36–39] In the case of outpatient elective catheterizations, which make up approximately half of greater than 600,000 PCI procedures performed annually in the United States, using TRA to facilitate efficient periprocedural care and SDD has resulted in enhanced patient satisfaction and cost savings.[19–22,36–42]

Evidence supports that a TRA approach is particularly beneficial in patients at higher bleeding risk, because bleeding is a costly complication associated with longer LOS. In an analysis of internal admission cost data compiled from 5 PCI centers, a TRA approach was performed in 17% of cases and was associated with decreased LOS (2.5 vs 3.0 days, P<.001), less bleeding (1.1% vs 2.4%, P = .002), and a total cost savings of $830 per admission (95% CI $296–$1,364, P<.001) when compared with TFA. There was no significant difference in procedural cost. Savings were greater in patients with higher bleeding risk, with a savings of $642 in those with low bleeding risk that increased to $1621 in those with higher bleeding risk.[36] These results were consistent with findings from a retrospective cohort analysis of patients undergoing 61,509 PCI procedures in the Premier database during a period of 2004 to 2009. In this study, TRA use was associated with decreased inpatient hospitalization cost of $553 ($11,736 vs $12,288, P = .033). This savings was driven by an average LOS that was 0.3 days shorter in TRA versus TFA. In addition, 20% of the savings was attributed to decreased bleeding complications, and as a result, it was proposed that cost savings of using TRA would be maximized in those with highest risk of bleeding.[37]

In addition, in a 2008 analysis, Rao and colleagues[38] demonstrated that bleeding severity was positively associated with increases in LOS, with LOS increasing from 5.4 days in patients with no bleeding to 16.4 days in the event of severe bleeding (P<.01). This increase in LOS was accompanied by an increase in cost from $14,282 in the case of no bleeding to $21,674 with mild bleeding, $45,798 with moderate bleeding, and $66,564 with severe bleeding (P<.01). After adjustment for baseline patient characteristics, investigators determined that each moderate or severe bleeding event increased hospitalization costs by $3770, and each transfusion event increased costs by $2,080, with LOS driving increased costs associated with complications. It was concluded that minimizing complications and LOS is key to lowering the cost of PCI.

In an analysis using NCDR CathPCI Registry and Medicare claims data to assess potential savings from various clinical pathways in PCI for both SDD and TRA, out of 279,987 PCI patients during 2009 to 2012, 5.3% of patients undergoing PCI were SDD and 9.0% of these cases were performed via TRA. In cost analysis of various pathways, the most cost-efficient pathway was using TRA with SDD costing $13,389, followed by using TFA with SDD at $13,913 (Table 1). TFA with non–same-day discharge (NSDD) was most costly at $17,076. SDD was associated with an adjusted cost-reduction of $3502 (95% CI $3486–$3902). Comparing TRA versus TFA costs, TRA utilization reduced adjusted hospitalization cost by $916 for all LOS included in the analysis (95% CI $778–$1035) (Table 2). Patients being discharged the same day were more likely to have undergone TRA versus TFA (13.5% vs 4.5%). It was found that replacing the common practice of TFA and NSDD with widespread adoption of TRA with default plans for SDD could result in a significant cost savings.[39]

Systematic implementation of SDD for elective PCI has been described as a potential strategy for improving fiscal value as well as increasing patient satisfaction.[40] It has been previously shown that patients prefer decreased LOS for catheterization. In 1 study, about half of surveyed patients reported discharge on the same day of elective PCI as a priority.[22,41] Furthermore, in an observational analysis of patients undergoing elective PCI, SDD patients were more likely to have undergone TRA compared with NSDD (42% vs 5%, $P<.001$). In total, more patients underwent TFA than TRA in both SDD and NSDD groups, but there was a marked increase in TRA utilization over time, with greater than 4-fold increase in the proportion of cases with radial access over a 2-year period (7% to 30%). Among SDD patients, 99.3% were "extremely satisfied" with being discharged the same day, and all these patients rated their overall care as "excellent care." At follow-up, these SDD patients had zero adverse outcome events of mortality, bleeding, or VASC requiring treatment, and there was no difference in acute kidney injury (AKI). SDD patients had significantly lower median total PCI cost with a 39% savings in total cost per procedure ($10,425 vs $17,135, $P<.0001$). After propensity score adjustment, SDD resulted in cost savings of $7331 per case (95% CI $4370–$10,292). Implementation of the patient-centered SDD program was projected to result in single-institutional savings of $1.8 million annually based on end-of-study SDD and PCI rate and volume estimates. Cost savings were realized across all categories of medical costs, but the bulk of the saved costs were owed to decreases in variable direct costs, including laboratory tests, medications, medical and surgical supplies, and physician and nursing expenses.[42]

Institutional-level savings were confirmed in a nationally representative analysis of 672,470 elective PCIs across 493 US hospitals in the Premier Healthcare Database.[40] In this analysis, the unadjusted rate of SDD was 9.1% of all cases, although this rate was adjusted to 3.5% after accounting for high levels of interhospital practice variation. The higher unadjusted rate suggested that a few larger centers performing large numbers of SDD procedures resulted in a skewing of the unadjusted rate. Investigators concluded that SDD was significantly more likely in institutions performing TRA approach 20.6% of the time (incidence rate ratio 1.45; 95% CI 1.40–1.50; $P<.001$). In the cost analysis, SDD was associated with an adjusted savings of $5128 (95% CI $5006–$5248) per procedure with highest savings in the areas of central supply and reduced room and board costs. These savings came without consequence to clinical outcomes, because SDD was not associated with a higher rate of rehospitalization for bleeding, AKI, or MI, and there was no difference in postdischarge mortality. The high rates

Table 1		
Adjusted costs of percutaneous coronary intervention by care pathway groups		
Care Pathway Group	**Adjusted PCI Cost ($)**	**95% CI ($)**
SDD	13,256	13,091–13,406
NSDD	16,753	16,673–16,833
TRA (SDD & NSDD)	15,786	15,642–15,928
TFA (SDD & NSDD)	16,701	16,620–16,787
TRA-SDD	13,389	13,161–13,607
TRA-NSDD	16,420	16,298–16,553
TFA-SDD	13,913	13,772–14,060
TFA-NSDD	17,076	16,999–17,147

Table 1 adapted with permission from Amin AP, Patterson M, House JA, et al. Costs Associated with Access Site and Same-Day Discharge Among Medicare Beneficiaries Undergoing Percutaneous Coronary Intervention: An Evaluation of the Current Percutaneous Coronary Intervention Care Pathways in the United States. JACC Cardiovasc Interv. 2017;10(4):342-351.

Table 2
Adjusted cost difference between care pathways

Care Pathway Group	Cost Difference ($)	95% CI ($)	P Value
TRA vs TFA	−916	−1035 to −778	<.001
SDD vs NSDD	−3502	−3648 to −3347	<.001
TRA SDD vs TRA NSDD	−3035	−3273 to −2825	<.001
TRA SDD vs TFA SDD	−527	−776 to −295	<.001
TRA SDD vs TFA NSDD	−3689	−3902 to −3486	<.001
TRA NSDD vs TFA SDD	2508	2324–2680	<.001
TRA NSDD vs TFA NSDD	−652	−765 to −534	<.001
TFA SDD vs TFA NSDD	−3160	−3299 to −3027	<.001

Table 2 adapted with permission from Amin AP, Patterson M, House JA, et al. Costs Associated with Access Site and Same-Day Discharge Among Medicare Beneficiaries Undergoing Percutaneous Coronary Intervention: An Evaluation of the Current Percutaneous Coronary Intervention Care Pathways in the United States. JACC Cardiovasc Interv. 2017;10(4):342-351.

of interhospital variation illustrated that institutional practices, rather than solely patient attributes, may influence the treatment one receives. This variation decreased over the 9-year study period, but during this time, there was a range of SDD rate that varied from as low as 0% to as high as 83%, and practice variability was still high at the conclusion of the study. These variations emphasize the importance of deliberate, data-driven implementations for successful and safe SDD programs. Nationwide utilization of such a program with SDD rates as observed in the top decile was projected to save the health care system approximately $577 million annually based on NCDR elective catheterization procedure volumes.[40]

BALANCING MEASURES OF TRANSRADIAL ACCESS

Although studies have identified several benefits associated with TRA, there are limitations that must be acknowledged. Data from randomized trials reveal that TRA has been linked to higher rate of procedure failure, need for crossover to femoral access, and greater fluoroscopy time.[9–13,43,44] In 1 study, radial artery spasm, subclavian tortuosity, and inadequate guide support were found to be the most common reasons for procedure failure.[45] However, although crossover from radial to femoral access is associated with reduced patient satisfaction, the absolute increase in procedure failure risk with TRA is only 4% higher than TFA (RR 0.97, 95% CI 0.96–0.98).[22,27] In addition, TRA is associated with a learning curve that must be overcome before realizing the benefits.[45] In less experienced operators, greater rates of failure

requiring crossover to femoral access, increased contrast use, and longer fluoroscopy time have been observed.[45] However, the learning curve is not prohibitive, and at a threshold of only 50 cases, failure rates approximate those of expert users.[45] Last, among operators who perform a high proportion of transradial cases, it has been proposed that a potential exists for greater rates of VASCs during femoral crossover: the "Campeau Radial Paradox."[46] However, in this study it is possible that the paradox existed because patients selected for femoral access had more comorbidities than those selected for radial access; in fact, there was a higher incidence of risk factors for major vascular complications in the femoral group.[46] Furthermore, a retrospective analysis of 235,250 TFA PCIs in the British Cardiovascular Intervention Society demonstrated no association between recent center femoral proportion or volume and femoral access site complications.[47] Nonetheless, this finding highlights the importance of maintaining skill sets in both radial and femoral access.

SUMMARY

In recent years, there has been growing adoption of TRA utilization for all types of cardiac catheterization with substantial evidence of safety, comfort, and economic advantages. In addition to reduced complications, particularly bleeding and vascular events, there are data demonstrating increased patient satisfaction, less pain and discomfort, earlier ambulation, and reduced LOS with TRA versus TFA. Furthermore, the substantial cost savings associated with TRA PCI through reduced complications and LOS underscore the potential for this technique to save millions in US health care costs. Although these advantages have been noted widely in the literature, there are challenges to realizing these benefits, including a steep operator learning curve, ability to gain and maintain experience in TRA and TFA, and practice variation between hospitals and operators. Overall, these data underscore the value of the radial approach for cardiac catheterization and PCI for improved patient safety, greater patient satisfaction, and substantially lower health care spending. There are few therapies in medicine that improve patient outcomes at a lower cost: TRA for PCI is one of the most robust examples.

REFERENCES

1. Campeau L. Percutaneous radial artery approach for coronary angiography. Cathet Cardiovasc Diagn 1989;16(1):3–7.
2. Kiemeneij F, Laarman GJ. Percutaneous radial artery approach for coronary stent implantation. Cathet Cardiovasc Diagn 1993;30(2):173–8.
3. Sewell WH. Coronary angiography by the Sones technique—technical considerations. Am J Roentgenol 1965;96:673–83.
4. Seldinger SI. Catheter replacement of the needle in percutaneous arteriography; a new technique. Acta Radiol 1953;39(5):368–76.
5. Judkins MP. Selective coronary arteriography. I. A percutaneous transfemoral technic. Radiology 1967;89(5):815–24.
6. Amplatz K, Formanek G, Stranger P, et al. Mechanics of selective coronary artery catheterization via femoral approach. Radiology 1967;89:1040–7.
7. Ryan TJ. The coronary angiogram and its seminal contributions to cardiovascular medicine over five decades. Circulation 2002;106(6):752–6.
8. Rao SV, Ou FS, Wang TY, et al. Trends in the prevalence and outcomes of radial and femoral approaches to percutaneous coronary intervention: a report from the National Cardiovascular Data Registry. JACC Cardiovasc Interv 2008;1:379–86.
9. Valgimigli M, Gagnor A, Calabró P, et al. Radial versus femoral access in patients with acute coronary syndromes undergoing invasive management: a randomised multicentre trial. Lancet 2015; 385(9986):2465–76.
10. Jolly SS, Yusuf S, Miemela K, et al. Radial versus femoral access for coronary angiography and intervention in patients with acute coronary syndromes (RIVAL): a randomised, parallel group, multicentre trial. Lancet 2011;377:1409–20.
11. Romagnoli E, Biondi-Zoccai G, Sciahbasi A, et al. Radial versus femoral randomized investigation in ST-segment elevation acute coronary syndrome: the RIFLE-STEACS (Radial Versus Femoral Randomized Investigation in ST-Elevation Acute Coronary Syndrome) study. J Am Coll Cardiol 2012; 60(24):2481–9.
12. Bernat I, Horak D, Strasek J, et al. ST-segment elevation myocardial infarction treated by radial or femoral approach in a multicenter randomized control trial: the STEMI-RADIAL trial. J Am Coll Cardiol 2014;63(10):964–72.
13. Rao SV, Hess CN, Barham B, et al. A registry-based randomized trial comparing radial and femoral approaches in women undergoing percutaneous coronary intervention: the SAFE-PCI for Women (Study of Access Site for Enhancement of PCI for Women) trial. JACC Cardiovasc Interv 2014;7(8):857–67.
14. Gutierrez A, Tsai TT, Stanislawski MA, et al. Adoption of transradial percutaneous coronary intervention and outcomes according to center radial volume in the Veterans Affairs Healthcare system: insights from the Veterans Affairs clinical assessment, reporting, and tracking (CART) program. Circ Cardiovasc Interv 2013;6(4):336–46.
15. Feldman DN, Swaminathan RJ, Kaltenbach, et al. Adoption of radial access and comparison of outcomes to femoral access in percutaneous coronary intervention an updated report from the National Cardiovascular Data Registry (2007–2012). Circulation 2013;127:2295–306.
16. NCDR–performance reports: using data to drive quality. Available at: https://cvquality.acc.org/NCDR-Home/reports. Accessed July 3, 2019.
17. Naidu SS, Aronow HD, Box LC, et al. SCAI expert consensus statement: 2016 best practices in the cardiac catheterization laboratory: (endorsed by the Cardiological Society of India, and Sociedad Latino Americana de Cardiologia Intervencionista; affirmation of value by the Canadian Association of Interventional Cardiology-Association Canadienne de Cardiologie d'Intervention). Catheter Cardiovasc Interv 2016;88(3):407–23.
18. Mason PJ, Shah B, Tamis-Holland JE, et al. An update on radial artery access and best practices for transradial coronary angiography and intervention in acute coronary syndrome: a scientific statement from the American Heart Association. Circ Cardiovasc Interv 2018;11(9):e000035.
19. Louvard Y, Lefèvre T, Allain A, et al. Coronary angiography through the radial or the femoral approach: the CARAFE study. Catheter Cardiovasc Interv 2001;52(2):181–7.
20. Cooper CJ, El-Shiekh RA, Cohen DJ, et al. Effect of transradial access on quality of life and cost of cardiac catheterization: a randomized comparison. Am Heart J 1999;138(3 Pt 1):430–6.
21. Ness CN, Krucoff MW, Sheng S, et al. Comparison of quality-of-life measures after radial versus femoral artery access for cardiac catheterization in

women: results of the study of access site for enhancement of percutaneous coronary intervention for women quality-of-life substudy. Am Heart J 2015;170(2):371–9.

22. Kok MM, Weernink MGM, von Birgelen C, et al. Patient preference for radial versus femoral vascular access for elective coronary procedures: the PREVAS study. Catheter Cardiovasc Interv 2018;91(1): 17–24.

23. Cantor WJ, Mehta SR, Yuan F, et al. Radial versus femoral access for elderly patients with acute coronary syndrome undergoing coronary angiography and intervention: insights from the RIVAL trial. Am Heart J 2015;170(5):880–6.

24. Alnasser SM, Bagai A, Jolly SS, et al. Transradial approach for coronary angiography and intervention in the elderly: a meta-analysis of 777,841 patients. Int J Cardiol 2017;228:45–51.

25. Hibbert B, Simard T, Wilson KR, et al. Transradial versus transfemoral artery approach for coronary angiography and percutaneous coronary intervention in the extremely obese. JACC Cardiovasc Interv 2012;5(8):819–26.

26. Ferrante G, Rao SV, Jüni P, et al. Radial versus femoral access for coronary interventions across the entire spectrum of patients with coronary artery disease: a meta-analysis of randomized trials. JACC Cardiovasc Interv 2016;9(14):1419–34.

27. Kolkailah AA, Alreshq RS, Muhammed AM, et al. Transradial versus transfemoral approach for diagnostic coronary angiography and percutaneous coronary intervention in people with coronary artery disease. Cochrane Database Syst Rev 2018;4: CD012318.

28. Ratib K, Mamas MA, Anderson SG, et al. Access site practice and procedural outcomes in relation to clinical presentation in 439,947 patients undergoing percutaneous coronary intervention in the United Kingdom. JACC Cardiovasc Interv 2015;8(1 Pt A):20–9.

29. American College of Cardiology 19 – 68th Annual Scientific Session & Expo – the SAFARI-STEMI trial slides. Available at: https://www.acc.org/~/media/Clinical/PDF-Files/Approved-PDFs/2019/03/15/ACC19_Slides/Mar18_Mon/1145amET_SAFARI-STEMI-acc-2019.pdf. Accessed July 3, 2019.

30. Reddy BK, Brewter PS, Walsh T, et al. Randomized comparison of rapid ambulation using radial, 4 French femoral access, or femoral access with AngioSeal closure. Catheter Cardiovasc Interv 2004;62(2):143–9.

31. Chodor P, Krupa H, Kurek T, et al. RADIal versus femoral approach for percutaneous coronary interventions in patients with Acute Myocardial Infarction (RADIAMI): a prospective, randomized, single-center clinical trial. Cardiol J 2009;16: 332–40.

32. Jaffe R, Hong T, Sharieff W, et al. Comparison of radial versus femoral approach for percutaneous coronary interventions in octogenarians. Catheter Cardiovasc Interv 2007;69(6):815–20.

33. Basu D, Singh PM, Tiwari A, et al. Meta-analysis comparing radial versus femoral approach in patients 75 years and older undergoing percutaneous coronary procedures. Indian Heart J 2017;69(5): 580–8.

34. Bundled payments for care improvement advanced (BPCI advanced). Centers for Medicare & Medicaid Services. Available at: https://innovation.cms.gov/initiatives/bpci-advanced. Accessed June 8, 2019.

35. Wadhera RK, Yeh RW, Joynt Maddox KE. The rise and fall of mandatory cardiac bundled payments. JAMA 2018;319(4):335–6.

36. Amin AP, House JA, Safley DM, et al. Costs of transradial percutaneous coronary intervention. JACC Cardiovasc Interv 2013;6(8):827–34.

37. Safley DM, Amin AP, House JA, et al. Comparison of costs between transradial and transfemoral percutaneous coronary intervention: a cohort analysis from the premier research database. Am Heart J 2013;165(3):303–9.e2.

38. Rao SV, Kaul PR, Liao L, et al. Association between bleeding, blood transfusion, and costs among patients with non-ST-segment elevation acute coronary syndromes. Am Heart J 2008;155(2):369–74.

39. Amin AP, Patterson M, House JA, et al. Costs associated with access site and same-day discharge among Medicare beneficiaries undergoing percutaneous coronary intervention: an evaluation of the current percutaneous coronary intervention care pathways in the United States. JACC Cardiovasc Interv 2017;10(4):342–51.

40. Amin AP, Pinto D, House JA, et al. Association of same-day discharge after elective percutaneous coronary intervention in the United States with costs and outcomes. JAMA Cardiol 2018;3(11): 1041–9.

41. Ziakas A, Klinke P, Fretz E, et al. Same-day discharge is preferred by the majority of the patients undergoing radial PCI. J Invasive Cardiol 2004;16(10):562–5.

42. Amin AP, Crimmins-Reda P, Miller S, et al. Novel patient-centered approach to facilitate same-day discharge in patients undergoing elective percutaneous coronary intervention. J Am Heart Assoc 2018;7(4) [pii:e005733].

43. Jolly SS, Cairns J, Niemela K, et al. Effect of radial versus femoral access on radiation dose and the importance of procedural volume: a substudy of the multicenter randomized RIVAL trial. JACC Cardiovasc Interv 2013;6:258–66.

44. Bradley SM, Rao SV, Curtis JP, et al. Change in hospital-level use of transradial percutaneous coronary intervention and periprocedural

outcomes: insights from the National Cardiovascular Data Registry. Circ Cardiovasc Qual Outcomes 2014;7(4):550–9.

45. Ball WT, Sharieff W, Jolly SS, et al. Characterization of operator learning curve for transradial coronary interventions. Circ Cardiovasc Interv 2011;4(4): 336–41.

46. Azzalini L, Tosin K, Chabot-Blanchet M, et al. The benefits conferred by radial access for cardiac catheterization are offset by a paradoxical increase in the rate of vascular access site complications with femoral access: the campeau radial paradox. JACC Cardiovasc Interv 2015;8(14):1854–64.

47. Hulme W, Sperrin M, Kontopantelis E, et al. Increased radial access is not associated with worse femoral outcomes for percutaneous coronary interventions in the United Kingdom. Circ Cardiovasc Interv 2017;10:e004279.

Moving?

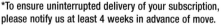

Make sure your subscription moves with you!

To notify us of your new address, find your **Clinics Account Number** (located on your mailing label above your name), and contact customer service at:

Email: journalscustomerservice-usa@elsevier.com

800-654-2452 (subscribers in the U.S. & Canada)
314-447-8871 (subscribers outside of the U.S. & Canada)

Fax number: 314-447-8029

Elsevier Health Sciences Division
Subscription Customer Service
3251 Riverport Lane
Maryland Heights, MO 63043

*To ensure uninterrupted delivery of your subscription, please notify us at least 4 weeks in advance of move.

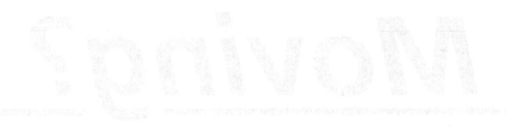

Printed and bound by CPI Group (UK) Ltd, Croydon, CR0 4YY

03/10/2024

01040371-0008